SECOND EDITION

# FOCUSED for SOCCER

## Bill Beswick

Human Kinetics

**Library of Congress Cataloging-in-Publication Data**

Beswick, Bill.
  Focused for soccer / Bill Beswick. -- 2nd ed.
    p. cm.
  Includes bibliographical references and index.
  ISBN-13: 978-0-7360-8411-6 (soft cover)
  ISBN-10: 0-7360-8411-8 (soft cover)
  1. Soccer--Psychological aspects. I. Title.
  GV943.9.P7B47 2010
  796.33401'9--dc22

                                     2010006723

ISBN-10: 0-7360-8411-8 (print)
ISBN-13: 978-0-7360-8411-6 (print)

The Web addresses cited in this text were current as of April 2010, unless otherwise noted.

**Acquisitions Editor:** Tom Heine; **Managing Editor:** Laura Podeschi; **Assistant Editor:** Steven Calderwood; **Copyeditor:** Mary Rivers; **Indexer:** Betty Frizzéll; **Permission Manager:** Martha Gullo; **Graphic Designer:** Bob Reuther; **Graphic Artist:** Julie L. Denzer; **Cover Designer:** Keith Blomberg; **Photographer (cover):** Clive Rose/Getty Images Sport; **Photo Asset Manager:** Laura Fitch; **Photo Production Manager:** Jason Allen; **Art Manager:** Kelly Hendren; **Associate Art Manager and Illustrator:** Alan L. Wilborn; **Printer:** Sheridan Books

Human Kinetics books are available at special discounts for bulk purchase. Special editions or book excerpts can also be created to specification. For details, contact the Special Sales Manager at Human Kinetics.

Printed in the United States of America     10  9  8  7  6  5  4  3  2  1

The paper in this book is certified under a sustainable forestry program.

**Human Kinetics**
Web site: www.HumanKinetics.com

*United States:* Human Kinetics
P.O. Box 5076
Champaign, IL 61825-5076
800-747-4457
e-mail: humank@hkusa.com

*Canada:* Human Kinetics
475 Devonshire Road Unit 100
Windsor, ON N8Y 2L5
800-465-7301 (in Canada only)
e-mail: info@hkcanada.com

*Europe:* Human Kinetics
107 Bradford Road
Stanningley
Leeds LS28 6AT, United Kingdom
+44 (0) 113 255 5665
e-mail: hk@hkeurope.com

*Australia:* Human Kinetics
57A Price Avenue
Lower Mitcham, South Australia 5062
08 8372 0999
e-mail: info@hkaustralia.com

*New Zealand:* Human Kinetics
P.O. Box 80
Torrens Park, South Australia 5062
0800 222 062
e-mail: info@hknewzealand.com

E4874

This second edition is dedicated to two of my brothers, Fred and Frank. It was Frank who persuaded me of the importance of getting a good education. Fred changed my life by buying me a membership at the Manchester YMCA for my 14th birthday. Fred's constant support and the opportunities provided by the YMCA have been significant factors in creating the momentum that shaped my life in sport.

Education and sport have been dominant and successful themes in my life, and for that I owe Fred and Frank my thanks.

# Contents

# Foreword

I first heard Bill speak when just starting out on my coaching career, and my experience as a player convinced me that Bill's message—the power of a positive attitude—was key in getting the best out of players and teams.

For the past 15 years, Bill has worked with me at a number of Premier League teams and with the England National Team. Together we developed a coaching philosophy that focuses on the physical, technical, and tactical qualities of teams, while always embracing the power of positive attitudes and making the right lifestyle choices.

Working alongside Bill, I have seen firsthand the powerful influence of an experienced sport psychologist creating a positive environment within the emotional rollercoaster of a Premier League season. This book contains many examples showing how the application of sport psychology has enhanced performance. I too have become more of a psychologist and less of a trainer in seeking to build and maintain winning teams.

With Bill as a mentor and colleague, I have become a better student of the game and an avid reader of books sharing the lessons and experiences of great coaches. All coaches—from grassroots to the professional level—must constantly advance their knowledge, and this book is key to their understanding of the mental side of the game.

Study, learn, and enjoy.

Steve McClaren
Head Coach, FC Twente (Holland)
Former England National Team Head Coach

# Preface

The first edition of this book was based on my experience as an international basketball coach and early work as an applied sport psychologist at Derby County FC in the English Premier League. The success of the book throughout the world emphasized that coaches felt the need to understand the application of psychology to soccer.

Since that time, my career in soccer has provided a much more extensive range of knowledge and experience. At Manchester United I could study a great manager, learn how to influence elite players, and examine the challenge of winning after winning. In comparison, at Middlesbrough FC as assistant manager, I came to understand how a team with a strong culture and positive attitudes, though less talented, could still win big games. At Sunderland AFC the thrust of my work was on getting the best out of players individually and motivating the team as a whole. Here, the performance of a team in the bottom half of the Premier League depended on maintaining a positive attitude and the ability to recover well from setbacks.

Being the first-ever sport psychologist appointed to work with the England senior men's team afforded experience of the challenge to produce consistent excellence in an environment under extreme scrutiny. Representative teams can lack continuity and stability, and the addition of very high expectations and the consequences of failure are factors that combine to create a context where performance anxiety is difficult to overcome.

So I have had a far richer experience to draw on for this second edition. Two topics deserved completely new chapters—The Power of Attitude: Developing a Winning Mind-Set and Coaching: Creating the Future. Other chapters have been completely refreshed, updated, and illustrated with new case studies. This time the material also reflects and benefits from experience assisting college coaches in the United States, including insights on the psychology of coaching female players.

Although the material is specific to soccer, the principles of human behavior are common to most sports, so this book has benefits for those involved in other sports too.

Whatever your gender, level, sport, or background, this book aims to interest and challenge. Your attitude is within your control, and you can improve your performance immediately and significantly by adopting the ideas and strategies in the following pages.

Bill Beswick

May 2010

# Acknowledgments

**M**y first and most grateful acknowledgment goes to all the players and coaches I have had the opportunity to work with in England, Europe, and the United States. We have learned many lessons together, and I thank them for our shared experiences.

Since writing the first edition, a number of coaches deserve particular mention for their forward-thinking approach to sport psychology and their commitment to working with me.

Steve McClaren is a coach who has consistently incorporated sport psychology into his philosophy—and included me in his coaching teams. The coaching team at Middlesbrough—Steve McClaren, Steve Harrison, Paul Barron, and Steve Round—was the best I have ever worked with, and my thanks go to them all.

I value enormously my opportunities to teach (and learn) in the United States, and among a number of great people and dedicated coaches, would pick out three who worked hard to make this happen—Mike Noonan (while at Brown University), Schellas Hyndman (FC Dallas and formerly Southern Methodist University), and Brent Erwin (Southern Methodist University).

Sportsmind is a team enterprise, so thanks are due to "the two Vals" (my wife and Val Holmes), who together keep me onside with their support. Similarly, thanks go to Tom Heine and Laura Podeschi, my guides and editors at Human Kinetics.

# CHAPTER 1

# The Power of Attitude: Developing a Winning Mind-Set

Champions must have both skill and will,
but the will must be stronger.

**Muhammad Ali, world champion boxer**

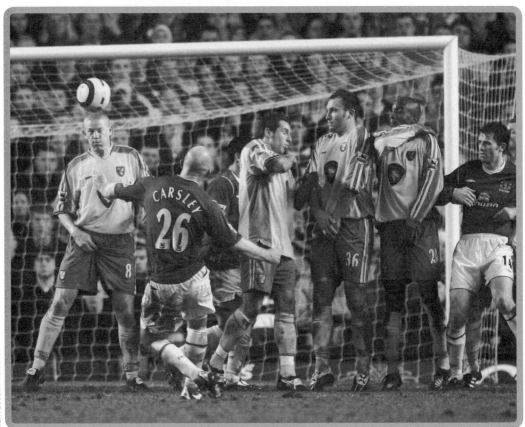

here are three kinds of athletes in this room. The first kind, the gods, are those blessed with both talent and attitude. They will succeed at the highest levels—unless coaches get in their way. The second kind have talent but poor attitude, and they are doomed to waste their potential, occasionally flattering to deceive, but more often letting themselves and others down. Finally, we have those with less talent but great attitude: athletes who will maximize every opportunity and whose commitment will often be rewarded by success in their sport. I probably don't need to point out that while your talent base might be difficult to improve, your attitude can change as much as you want and when you want.

With these words, spoken to the student athletes of Brown University, I underlined the importance and power of attitude to the pursuit of excellence in sport. I believe that playing soccer well is a combination of talent and attitude. Such combinations vary from player to player, field position to field position, and situation to situation. There are many critical career points in the development of a player, and at each stage, success is possible only if both talent and attitude can meet the new demands.

Talent, of course, is important in establishing the limits of potential, but it is only a starting point. As John Wooden, the great basketball coach, said, "Talent gets you to the door; character takes you inside."

Since 1995, I have been the team psychologist to both English Premier League soccer clubs and England National soccer teams. In every situation, I have worked with the coaches and players to maximize the power of positive attitude. Each season, I see examples of what can be achieved when players and teams get their attitudes right:

■ An underachieving young player, Lee Carsley, let his negative attitude get in the way of his physical and technical potential. After a short program of attitude change, Lee won the battle with his inner self, and positive attitudes replaced negative attitudes. His newfound mental toughness led to a highly successful Premier League career with Derby County, Blackburn, Everton, and Birmingham.

■ A poll of coaches at the start of a season ranked Derby County 18th of 20 teams in the Premier League in terms of talent. Yet with less talent, Derby finished that year in 7th position! The difference between projected and actual ranking was the result of consistent coaching for positive attitude and, equally important, always treating setbacks as an opportunity for renewed learning.

■ The Manchester United team was a goal down in the European Cup final when the referee signaled three minutes of extra time. As they waited to defend a corner, the United players saw the cup being brought into the stadium decorated with Bayern Munich colors. Anger and renewed determination led to a two-goal response by United and victory!

■ For the eighth time in their 128-year history, the Middlesbrough Football Club reached a cup final. But they had lost their previous seven finals, which put them in a situation where overtraining and overcoaching were tempting. The coaches decided to be brave and "try easy." After a relaxed and fun week of preparation, the team scored twice in the opening seven minutes of the game and went on to win Middlesbrough's first-ever trophy.

■ The England team, struggling with form and injuries, had to face world champion Brazil in front of 90,000 spectators and a worldwide TV audience to reopen the renovated Wembley Stadium. With only three days to prepare, the coaches made attitude their number one priority and set out to build confidence and mental toughness. A determined England team, led by their courageous captain, John Terry, gained a 1-1 draw after leading with two minutes to go.

■ Chris Riggott, a Premier League player, lost his confidence and motivation after an injury and subsequent nonselection. After a short meeting, when he was advised to take responsibility for his attitude and change it from negative to positive, he returned to his club with renewed mental toughness. Four days later Chris was recalled into the first team and won the MVP award in a nationally televised game.

■ Sunderland, new to the Premier League, made up for their talent deficit with a wonderful team spirit. Their determined attitude resulted in five key wins, achieved when they scored the deciding goals in the few minutes of extra time added on by the referee at the end of the game.

■ Paul Robinson, England's goalkeeper, conceded a goal to Croatia in an important away game when a back pass bobbled over his foot as he attempted to kick clear. England lost the game, and everybody understood that Paul would face relentless criticism from fans and the media. I waited in the locker room until the manager had finished his postgame talk and then made my way over to Paul. He waved me away, saying, "I cannot always choose the situation I am in, but I can always choose my response." Paul's attitude was mature, professional, and dignified; he and everybody else recovered and moved on.

In each of these cases, success was based on a positive mental attitude combined with the hard work of effective preparation. Each team mentioned here believed they could win any game on any given day. This was especially true when the team was the underdog, and the power of great attitude could provide the winning edge. Each of these players found success by getting control of his mental and emotional state and then letting this winning attitude drive his performance.

# Understanding Attitude

Attitude is the translation into action of a player's thoughts and feelings. Players think, feel, and then act, in that order. Soccer challenges the players' thoughts and feelings, and often success is doing what it takes in spite of their fears.

A winning attitude will be reflected by action signs such as these:

- Physical intensity
- Great mental focus
- High emotional energy
- Mental toughness and resilience

Performance potential may be limited by talent, but attitude is the driving force to achievement. As the well-known basketball coach Bobby Knight once stated, "Don't give me players who want to win—give me players who want to prepare to win."

Coaches judge individual or team attitudes by the behavior they see on and around the soccer field. Good coaches are great observers and will be tuned to behaviors that indicate a player's state of mind. I remember

## Yasmin's Story

One of the best examples I have of performance following attitude concerns a 14-year-old soccer player from Liverpool. Yasmin was captain of her school team when they reached the Liverpool Schools Cup Final—a big occasion! After a tough 90 minutes, the score was 0-0, and extra time—very tiring for young players—did not produce a winner.

The referee called both captains aside and offered a penalty shoot-out but recommended they share the cup six months each. Yasmin's teammates were so tired they all wanted to share the cup; the goalkeeper was in tears at the thought of a penalty shoot-out. After consulting with their teammates, the captains reported back to the referee, and Yasmin's opponent requested sharing the cup. Yasmin asked for a penalty shoot-out, but when she returned to her team, she told them it was their opponents who had selected the shoot-out! Yasmin took the first penalty shot, scored, and then, switching places with her team's goalkeeper, she saved the first three spot kicks, winning the game for her team.

When interviewed afterward, Yasmin explained her actions: "I only dream of winning cups, not sharing them."

holding back a head coach from a verbal assault on a young player whose performance on the training field was unfocused and careless. One water break later, we learned that the player's parents had split up the night before, and he wasn't sure where home was anymore. All the clues are there if coaches learn to observe.

The attitude that players bring to practice or game day reflect three main influences:

**1.** Each player has a unique personality that shapes the way he sees the world—for example, as an optimist or pessimist, introvert or extrovert, fighter or victim.

**2.** Each player's attitude is influenced by the significant people in his life. These will include parents, guardians, peer groups, and coaches. If the player is successful and progresses through competitive levels of soccer, this group will grow and diversify, adding business agents, media personnel, and personal trainers.

**3.** A player's attitude is also shaped by the coaching and playing environment he finds himself in. A player is more likely to be positive, enthusiastic, and committed if these elements are in place:

– He has good coaches.

– He trains and plays in great facilities.

When a performance problem is attitudinal and not physical or technical, coaches should know the key questions to ask:

● Is the problem the player's personality?
● Is the player being influenced negatively by the people around him?
● Is this related to a coaching or playing problem?

One of the great dangers facing young and talented performers is that success comes easily, and the importance of developing attitude is ignored. Ed Smith, English cricket player and author, recognized this problem: "Super-talented young sportsmen, never having needed resilience thus far, often lack the psychological capacity to develop it when life gets tough in the big leagues" (2008, 45).

Coaches of young players must always find patience and time for the late developers who will probably have their attitude in place when their talent emerges. Early defeats can lead to subsequent victories. Many observers of Michael Jordan's talent believe that being cut from his high school team was the foundation for the determination that took him to the top.

A player's (or team's) attitude is defined by his response to the challenge he sees before him. A positive mental attitude can be defined as a constructive response to stress. If a player's definition of the situation is

- I am familiar with this challenge,
- I have successfully dealt with this before,
- I am fully prepared for it now, and
- I am excited by the chance to prove myself,

it is probable that his attitude will drive his talent to success.

If the reverse is true—the player or team doubts his ability to meet the challenge—then a negative attitude will probably precipitate failure. The hardest questions a soccer player asks are the ones he asks himself. In the examples shown at the start of this chapter, both Lee Carsley and Chris Riggott had to answer this question: "What am I willing to do to become a successful soccer player?"

So the starting point of performance effectiveness is the player or team's definition of the situation based on perceptions of preparedness. Coaches who prepare their teams well are far more likely to develop winning attitudes.

When I started work as a sport psychologist, I believed that most performance and behavior issues would come from the player themselves, so I focused on one-on-one counseling. What I found was that players often became upset about the behavior of the head coach or the coaching staff or issues concerning their general coaching environment. Now I focus first on supporting the head coach and the staff and creating a good practice and playing environment, and then I deal with one-on-one player issues.

In their book *Catch Them Being Good,* Tony DiCicco and Colleen Hacker emphasize the importance of a supportive environment to female soccer players.

> Coaches and parents have to realize that their words, their body language and the way they present feedback is going to have an impact on performance. Negativity is antivision. Instead of building towards a positive vision, it tears it down, yielding ineffective and inappropriate coaching or parenting. (2002, 104)

To help players take responsibility for their attitude and learn to develop good mental habits, coaches could distribute the following key messages found in the sidebar on the following page, urging their players to keep them in a place where they can see them every day.

## Performance Follows Attitude

Thus a player or team's attitude derives from how he perceives each soccer situation he faces. For all human beings faced with a challenge, the choice is fight or flight, and successful soccer players must be the ones

## DEVELOPING POSITIVE MENTAL ATTITUDES: KEY MESSAGES

**1.** I believe in myself.

**2.** My self-talk will always be positive.

**3.** I will come to compete every day.

**4.** I will not surrender.

**5.** I will not turn against myself during tough times.

**6.** I cannot choose what is happening around me, but I can (and will) choose how I respond.

**7.** I will use setbacks as learning opportunities.

**8.** I will focus on my strengths and contain my weaknesses.

**9.** I understand that my role as a team member is to help my teammates win.

**10.** I will not come in second best to myself.

*There's a choice you make in everything you do. And you must always keep in mind The choice you make makes you!*

**Dr. Rob Gilbert, sport psychologist (2006, 36)**

who choose fight. Once that choice is made, a chain reaction takes place, coordinating mind and body:

- Our state of mind accepts the challenge (the confidence of preparation).
- Our emotions become positive drivers (excitement, determination).
- Our bodies prepare for action (high energy levels).
- We are resilient enough to handle setbacks (mental toughness).

Thus, we are in the best position to succeed with our actions.

So a positive attitude not only supplies the fuel for explosive and sustained performance but also shapes the player's capacity to build the range of mental skills required for coping with the challenge of soccer, a fact constantly reinforced in the literature of sport psychology.

Positive thinking leads to mental toughness, which in turn leads to the winning edge. Figure 1.1 (page 8) shows the journey to success where the player's talent base must be built upon by developing key mental qualities. Note that weaknesses shown at any stage can lead to rejection.

The key, therefore, is influencing players to think positively, producing a high and positive emotional state that says, "I really want to win," and thus creating high and positive energy levels.

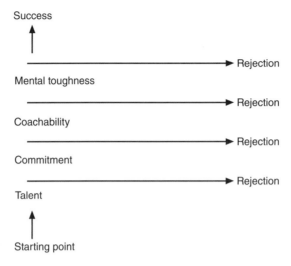

FIGURE 1.1 The player's journey to success.

# Staying Positive

The real battle in soccer is the internal drama fought between a player's strong side, "I can," versus a player's weak side, "I can't." Everyone who plays soccer faces a whole range of potential fears: fear of failing, doing something embarrassing, getting hurt, losing control, letting the team down, and not meeting expectations. The key fear is that player inadequacies will be discovered. If such internal fears are not dealt with, they can lead to negative player or team mind-sets and a state of anxiety about future events, a "what if?" fear that will inhibit performance. Because of this constant challenge to attitude and mental strength, the player is constantly open to positive or negative influences (see figure 1.2).

A team's collective mental state is determined by their response to the soccer challenge they are facing at any particular moment. Situations, people, and events all interconnect to influence mental state. Factors that can either be negative or positive, depending on the quality of the coach, are purpose, trust, change, conflict, distractions, setbacks, and environment. The team members individually or in small groups appraise the challenge ahead of them in relation to their perception of their resources. They mentally assess the strength of their opponents and match it against such factors as their own team selection, level of preparation, confidence in the coach, importance of the game, and whether the game is home or away.

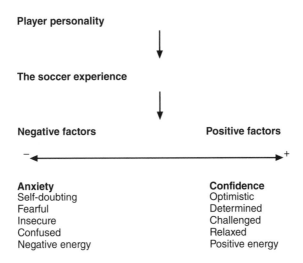

**Player personality**

**The soccer experience**

**Negative factors**                           **Positive factors**

−  ⟵─────────────────────⟶  +

**Anxiety**                                    **Confidence**
Self-doubting                                  Optimistic
Fearful                                        Determined
Insecure                                       Challenged
Confused                                       Relaxed
Negative energy                                Positive energy

FIGURE 1.2   Player attitude and mental strength.

## Shaping Team Thinking to Produce a High-Energy Performance

Middlesbrough was in crisis, having lost four games in a row. During the previous game at home, when we lost 4-0, a fan had run across the pitch and thrown his season tickets in the face of the manager, Steve McClaren.

The really bad news was that our next game was also at home to Chelsea, the league leaders. Before the match, I watched the players in the dressing room; it was clear from all the signs that the team had moved from confidence to anxiety (and some to a state of fear). At the coaches' meeting, a pregame speech based on tactics and strategy was discussed. I intervened and suggested the team needed a motivational speech. Steve agreed and asked me to quickly put something on paper. He presented it to the team beautifully:

> It's not the best team that wins football matches but the best team on that day. You can be the best team today. All you have to do is want it more than they do. You have won big games before, so you know you can do it, and you know what it takes. You have to work harder, out-tackle them, outfight them, take the injuries, play through pain, show them you will do whatever it takes to win. And when you come back in here after 94 minutes, not a single one of you will have any regrets. So let's make it our day. Good luck!

We won 3-0 in the biggest upset of the season.

The following are possible outcomes:

1. Confidence: The team believes their resources outmatch their opponents'—"We should win."
2. Anxiety: The team believes their resources are fewer than their opponents'—"We might lose."
3. A combination of 1 and 2: The team is quite confident they have the resources to win but still see the opponent as a very real threat—the optimal performance state (see figure 1.3).

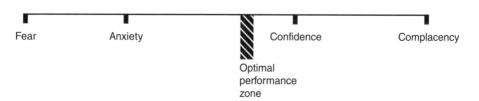

FIGURE 1.3 Optimal performance zone.

Players and teams can move frequently on the continuum between confidence and anxiety, both before and during the game. Coaches must be constantly aware of the battle between positives and negatives. A mentally strong, winning mind-set helps the player or team, assisted by the coach, stay positive and deal with the negatives that come their way, rather than just react to them. They may even learn to turn negatives into positives.

Coaches must watch for early negative signs at every training session and match. If coaches are too involved in the Xs and Os of tactics, they may not observe the players as people, as well as performers, and they could easily miss the early signs of a player in trouble. Great coaches are great observers and know how to look out for a decline in these things:

- Motivation
- Quality of practice
- Enthusiasm
- Communication
- Humor
- Discipline
- Voluntary extra work

They also know to look for an increase in these things:

- Placing blame
- Minor injuries
- Excuses
- Conflict
- Off-the-field issues

Coaches can also help players monitor their own attitude state by asking them to complete an attitude check such as the one in table 1.1.

| TABLE 1.1—Player Attitude Check |
|---|
| • Do you believe you can be a good player? |
| • Do you still know why? |
| • Have you set personal targets for the season? |
| • Are you still willing to pay the price? |
| • Are you taking care of your physical state? |
| • Are you a continual learner? |
| • Do you handle setbacks well? |
| • Do you deal with stress without losing control? |
| • Do you maintain your personal standards? |
| • Do you accept responsibility rather than blame others? |
| • Is soccer still fun? |

# Attitude Killers

Two great killers of player or team attitude exist. The first is expectations. As a player progresses, so do the expectations that he places on himself and faces from other people. Players, especially younger players, worry about what people will say about them, and they worry about what people will think about them. I have seen firsthand how the labeling of a young player as talented becomes a burden. In a chapter entitled "The Curse of Talent," Ed Smith quotes the English writer Cyril Connolly: "Whom the gods wish to destroy they first call promising" (2008, 43).

The second great attitude killer is consequences. The higher the level, the more players are reminded of the consequences of defeat, and the more they will face the internal battles of anxiety versus confidence, tension versus relaxation, and pressure versus pleasure.

It is the prime responsibility of the coach to relieve players of these burdens so that they may play with a winning attitude. The great coaches can get their players intense without getting them tense, a quality Luiz Felipe Scolari showed in guiding a very relaxed but focused Brazil to World Cup victory: "My priority is to ensure that my players feel more amateur than professional—they like the game, love it, do it with joy" (Smith 2008, 19).

Coaches must reframe these attitude killers in their players' minds with such messages as these:

■ The only expectations that are important are yours, those belonging to the others in this room, and what we decide to aim for as a team. Care a little less about what other people will think and say about you, and learn to act confidently.

■ Identify the worst that can happen and ask, "Can we deal with it?" It's OK to be worried—everybody worries—but you can act confidently regardless of how you feel. As a team, we will handle defeats together and use them as feedback in our journey to excellence.

In this way the coach takes responsibility for expectations and consequences and takes the pressure off the players. Coach Dean Smith, former
University of North Carolina basketball coach, dealt with winning by
praising his players for their efforts and losing by accepting that he could
have done a better job.

# Coaching for Attitude

If attitude is part of the winning equation for players, then clearly it must
be a priority for coaches. Coaches who want to win will recruit players
with both talent and attitude and shape their program of preparation to
consistently reinforce positive, winning attitudes. The modern coach will
become a little more of a psychologist and a little less of a trainer.

A coach who can positively shape a player's state of mind has a significant advantage in producing better performances. This is especially true
over the course of a league season where there will always be pressures
driving players to negative thinking. The key, therefore, is to influence
players to think positively—"I really want to win"—and thus produce high
and positive energy levels.

However, in the challenging roller coaster of a soccer league season,
attitudes can change every day. One day a player is a winner—in the game,
playing well, and healthy. The next day the player feels like a loser—out
of the game (benched), not playing well, or injured. There will be some
players in each squad who are "parked"—neither winners nor losers—and
swing between positive and negative attitudes.

Influencing attitude is a daily task, and every coach must develop a
toolbox of strategies for creating and maintaining the optimal attitude state
for both individual players and the team. The starting point for each coach
is to work from the end backward and to ask himself the key questions
for his particular situation (age, gender, level of competition, and so on):

- What is the ideal attitude state for my team as they run on the field?
- What can I do to create it?
- How would I recognize a negative attitude?
- What do I do (or not do) that creates negativity?
- What strategies do I have for moving players back from negative to
  positive?

Table 1.2 offers some elements of a winning attitude. In players blessed
with good attitude, most of these elements are already present, which is
why recruiters must check attitude. However, for the majority of players,

| TABLE 1.2—Performance Readiness: Elements of a Winning Attitude | |
|---|---|
| **Belief** | We can win. |
| **Commitment** | We will work hard to win for the whole 90 minutes. |
| **Confidence** | We are well prepared, understand our own jobs, and know what to do in each phase of the game. |
| **Focus** | We can exclude distractions and concentrate on the game. |
| **Discipline** | We understand the game plan and will carry it out. |
| **Freedom** | If we see something that might work, we are free to use our instincts because the coach will forgive positive mistakes. |
| **Bravery** | I will still want the ball when the game is on the line. |
| **Relaxed readiness** | We have prepared well, so we can be intense but not tense, play with smiles on our faces, and enjoy the game. |
| **Mental toughness** | We will come off the field with 11 players having won the game. |

some help is needed, and there will always be moments in long and challenging seasons when teams need an attitude check.

Table 1.3 (page 14) describes an exercise that will help players become more self-aware and understand the link between their mental state and its impact on their feelings, energy, and performance. Players should select their best and worst games in the recent past and try to recall the factors involved and whether there were any significant incidents. Often a low-energy performance can produce conflict, a lack of discipline, and so on; a high-energy performance can produce extraordinary moments and actions.

When the exercise is completed, players, with the help of their coaches, should be able to decide whether their attitude determined their performance, or their performance determined their attitude.

Coaches, therefore, have to come to terms with their power and ability to influence player attitude. Coaches must understand the following:

■ The personality of each player, his motivation, and how his attitude is best influenced (for instance, with praise or criticism). Coaches should look at their players in terms of their self-belief, commitment, mental toughness, and social ability to be part of a team. The younger the player, the more I recommend coaches have a good look at the parents for clues to the likely personality of the child. A better understanding of each player's personality is a step-by-step process that includes these elements:

## TABLE 1.3—A Player's Pregame Mental State and Its Impact on Performance

| | Best game | Worst game |
|---|---|---|
| Pregame mental state: "How was I thinking?" | | |
| Emotions: "How was I feeling?" | | |
| Energy levels: "What were my energy levels throughout the match?" | | |
| Performance level: "What words would describe my performance?" | | |
| Significant events: "Were there any particular actions that reflected my mental and emotional states?" | | |

From B. Beswick, 2010, *Focused for Soccer, Second Edition* (Champaign, IL: Human Kinetics).

- One-on-one communication
- Building a player fact file of relevant information both on and off the field
- Being more aware of the influence of players' families and friends
- Profiling the players' performance behavior, including mental, emotional, and lifestyle issues (see examples in chapter 2)

■ **Their own influence on player attitudes.** The actions of a coach are significant to player attitude. To be able to influence the player, the coach must win his respect and become a primary role model, setting an example in attitudes and behavior. One key factor is whether the coach is an optimist or pessimist—who would want to play for a pessimist?

I regularly conduct attitude "health checks" on soccer clubs, and very often the problems of attitude stem from the coaches themselves. Coaches who are tough but warm and forever optimistic can produce great results in the worst of circumstances. Arsene Wenger, manager of Arsenal Football Club, is an excellent example of a tough coach who knows exactly how he wants his team to play but also embraces positive and caring relationships that make players want to play for him and stay at Arsenal. Arsene is very aware of the impact of his personality. As he has stated, "The face of the coach is the mirror to the health of the team."

■ **How to drive their players to full achievement of their potential.** The secret, of course, is to manage this through disciplined and purposeful practice while at the same time creating an enjoyable coaching environment and showing the players that they are cared for as individuals.

■ **How to build a team and create player leadership that can exert positive peer pressure and reinforce winning attitudes.** Coaches should not underestimate the power of a positive locker room to set collective standards and bring players with problems into line.

■ **The impact of other significant people who influence their players**—parents, friends, agents, fans, media—and make these part of the solution and not the problem.

■ **The impact of the coaching and playing environment and how positive scenarios bring positive responses.** For younger players, the image and identity of their team are significant in peer group approval. Coaches can shape the coaching environment in these ways:

- Careful planning and preparation, thereby reducing organizational errors
- Constantly upgrading facilities and equipment
- Creating a resonant environment that recognizes and takes care of players' feelings

If a coach fully understands these influences on a player's attitudes and behavior, he has a vital start to understanding why specific problems may occur with individual players.

Coaches can also help shape player attitudes by creating a positive training and game environment. In particular, coaches can do the following:

■ Set performance goals as well as outcome goals. The team is challenged to win, but each player has some specific goals with which his performance may be assessed. Even in losing situations, it is important that players strive to meet their goals and that their coaches recognize when they have. One performance goal that often leads to winning is staying in the game regardless of the score. As U.S. football coach Paul "Bear" Bryant used to tell his team, "Winning isn't imperative, but getting tougher in the fourth quarter is."

■ Stress process, not outcome. When coaches focus on excellence rather than the scoreboard, players tend to relax more and focus on their own game, losing some of the fear of the outcome. Many games are lost because coaches were focused on winning while their opponents were focused on playing soccer well. For our first year at Middlesbrough (a team with low self-esteem and a definite problem with expectations and consequences), we only showed film clips of the team playing the game well. As mental toughness increased, we moved on to greater accountability.

■ Be bigger than the game. When a coach can be emotionally unbalanced by any one result, there is always a reflected pressure on his players. Great coaches take that pressure away by being, acting, and looking bigger than any one result. The coach will be disappointed by a defeat and will let the players know that, but he will not become pessimistic, blame individuals, or lose his sense of the bigger picture. Coaches have to take soccer seriously and care but not to the extent that defeats break their hearts.

After a winning streak of 12 games, Jim Smith, the former manager of Derby County, acknowledged his team's physical and mental fatigue. We discussed his reaction to the possibility of defeat. The following Saturday we lost an away game 5-0. Jim walked into the locker room and said, "That was a great run of wins, and I am proud of you. But now it is over, so let's come back in Monday ready to start a new run."

Finally, I would also warn coaches of the negative effects on attitude of overtraining and overcoaching. I understand that the majority of coaches do not get the opportunity to overtrain—they rarely see enough of their players. But for those who do—for example, college or professional coaches—the temptation to overtrain is ever present. Their task is balancing the very real and urgent need they feel to make sure every detail is covered against the possibility of draining their players physically and mentally. I have had real and painful experience with a head coach's demand for last-minute preparations that kill team attitude and leave "game legs" on the practice field. To quote Carol Heiss Jenkins, Olympic champion figure skater,

> You can want it too much;
> You can try too hard. (Gilbert 2006, 16)

Overcoaching—coaches telling players all they know rather than what the players can handle—is often the province of the young coach who wants to impress. Coaches who overcoach leave players confused and with an attitude that moves from confidence to anxiety. Simplicity, clarity, and appropriateness are the key checks for the coach who wishes to avoid overcoaching.

## Attitude and Female Players

In my experience, coaching female players calls for some unique skills. Although the same principles of building a winning attitude apply to both male and female players, there are some different emphases. I love the response of Mia Hamm, the great American player, when asked how she wanted to be coached: "Coach us like men, treat us like women" (DiCicco et al. 2002, 11).

Former U.S. women's national team coach Tony DiCicco added this:

> I believe, in order to create a new model of the champion, we must combine the best qualities of women with the best qualities of men. If we do, we will come up with an incredible athlete who is aggressive, tough, intense, assertive, fit, and competitive and finds a way to win while being relational, empathetic, compassionate and caring. (12)

So soccer behavior is not gender specific, but it is undoubtedly gender related. In my experience, coaches of female players may need to focus more on these elements:

- Building self-belief
- Defeating anxiety
- Dealing positively with mistakes and setbacks
- Dealing with success—fear of raised expectations
- Taking responsibility
- Handling relationship issues—teammates and coaches

Kathleen DeBoer, former professional basketball player and volleyball coach, examined gender and competition and had this to say: "Females value attachment, intimacy, and interdependence. Females fear rejection, isolation, and abandonment. They equate these conditions with loneliness and failure" (2004, 25).

She also understands that sports emphasize consequences—win or lose—and this presents a potential source of anxiety for female players: "The primacy of consequence, the very feature that makes competition appealing to males, makes it difficult for females" (27).

Coaches of women's teams need to be aware of these differences and understand the process by which their players reach a fully competitive and winning mind-set.

Figure 1.4 shows this process as it develops in three stages.

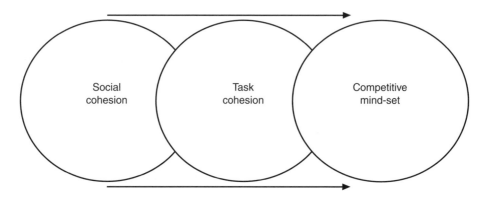

FIGURE 1.4 Building a winning attitude in female players.

## Stage 1: Social Cohesion

The starting point for most females in sport is emotional connection. Women need to feel socially included, safe, and cared for in order to best focus on winning. As Kathleen DeBoer explains,

> Girls come to the gym seeking to bond as the means to success; boys battle to achieve the same thing. Women enter a workplace predisposed to connect to achieve goals; men compete to achieve goals. Both want to win and both want results, but they both hold markedly different ideas on how to access their aspirations. Coaches must build a social contract with their teams that holds true regardless of results or setbacks—"we love you, win or lose." (2004, 17)

Anson Dorrance, soccer coach to the University of South Carolina women's team, tells the story of how he brought in a conditioning expert to take the warm-up. This worked out well physically—the players were always ready to practice—but not in terms of morale. Anson decided to return to his old warm-up where the girls chatted while jogging and stretching. This start allowed the opportunity for conversation, helping the players to share and build relationships. Anson realized team building had to begin with strong social cohesion.

Relationship coaching—caring for the players as people as well as athletes—is important to modern players but especially modern female players. Coaches have to reassure their female players that their relationship is secure regardless of the outcome of the match. Get the relationships right, and coaches will be surprised at the competitive power within female players and teams.

### Stage 2: Task Cohesion

Once social cohesion is in place, the coach can focus on helping the female players understand and take responsibility for their actions on the field. It is safe now to challenge players' attitudes and begin to increase mental toughness. However, coaches should remember that clarity and simplicity are key to task cohesion for both male and female players; and they must help their players understand their specific role, the game plan, and what they will be held accountable for.

### Stage 3: Competitive Mind-Set

Having worked through the first two stages and thus established the positive attitudes and relationships, coaches can now challenge the players to tough it out in the game. This attitude state includes wanting to compete and win, being assertive and aggressive, coping with setbacks, dealing with being star players, and being willing to step up and offer team leadership. Even then, coaches must be socially aware and maintain strong inclusive relationships.

This competitive mind-set can easily be destroyed if the coach does not understand after a defeat that their female players may feel guilt and need reassurance and rebonding quickly. Coaches must be careful to

- not hurt,
- not personalize,
- help generate realistic but positive feelings, and
- set a forward agenda with hope and optimism.

# 10 Steps to Building Winning Attitude

Now that we have established the power of attitude on performance for both male and female players, coaches need to identify strategies that reinforce that process. My experience recommends the following:

***Step 1: Recruit the right players.*** Recruit players with the character to win and a track record of commitment and success. In addition to looking at players in successful clubs, check the better players in losing teams;

they may have the stronger character. Try to get at least three character references, including a lifestyle appraisal, along with a more objective evaluation of physical, technical, and tactical talent.

***Step 2: Be the model for the attitude you want.*** Players, especially younger players, take their behavior lead from their coaches and often imitate their actions. So it is important that coaches model the attitudes and behavior they expect from the players, especially when times are difficult. Coaches should also surround their players with positive adults—assistant coaches, trainers, administrators, parents—who encourage the drive to excellence while offering a warm, supportive environment.

***Step 3: Create an inspirational vision.*** Soccer is the stuff of dreams, and coaches can create an enormous amount of attitude and energy if they are able to inspire. As Napoleon said, "Leaders deal in hope." Good coaches work every day to give their players a reason why it is important and worthwhile to maintain a positive and optimistic attitude. Coaches should work from the desired end backward and paint a picture for the players of how much they can achieve if they commit to the journey. Many coaches make the mistake of believing this is just a start-of-the-year exercise, but players need constant reminding, and every so often coaches should hold a quick meeting (on the field is okay) outlining these points, which is an approach of shared ownership and constant communication:

- Remember where *we* are going.
- This is where *we* are now.
- This is what *we* need to do.
- And this is why I believe together *we* can do it.

***Step 4: Give purpose and direction every day.*** Coach John Wooden always recommended that coaches should "make every day a masterpiece" and underlined that the practice session is the key to building mental as well as physical excellence. Players respond positively to well-planned, well-organized, and well-coached practice sessions that have challenges, learning, interest, and variety. It is in the everyday adaptation to the stress and competitive challenge of a well-planned session that players build positive winning attitudes. Coaches must set individual goals for their players as well as offer them the best competitive challenges every time they come to practice.

***Step 5: Coach the complete player.*** The profile of each player is a combination of talent and attitude, and while coaches operate through the development of talent—physical, technical, and tactical—they must not ignore the building of attitude. Ensuring the development of winning attitudes is not a classroom exercise but rather runs parallel to the players' response to the daily competitive challenges they must face and overcome.

Physical and mental development go hand in hand; and coaches must see beyond the function of a drill and appreciate the commitment, focus, decision making, and resilience involved.

***Step 6: Teach responsibility.***   A key element of a winning attitude is the player's ability to take responsibility for actions on and off the field. Once coaches have spent time with each player teaching a particular job in the team's tactical formation, they must take a step back and expect the player to take responsibility. Too many coaches struggle with trusting their players—and living with their mistakes—and thus deny them an opportunity to mature and build a powerful intrinsic motivation. The great players self-manage much of their development, and coaches should begin this process from an early age.

***Step 7: Encourage player leadership and peer group pressure.***   Finding player leadership is not easy these days, but coaches must work to give players the chance to offer positive leadership to their teammates. When one such individual is not available, I recommend coaches develop a core group of player leaders who can set a positive tone in the locker room and on the field. There is no doubt that the presence or absence of positive peer group pressure has a profound effect on player and team attitude.

***Step 8: Deal with setbacks well.***   Soccer is learned through trial and error: There will always be mistakes, setbacks, and defeats. Players need an environment of psychological safety if they are to build the courage to make things happen on the field. Nothing destroys this quicker than a coach out of control. Coaches must develop the emotional intelligence to deal with setbacks calmly and thoughtfully and not react emotionally. This mature sense of control will pass from coach to players and ensure that setbacks do not damage player attitude. Coaches must teach that failure, while disappointing, offers valuable feedback and a positive learning opportunity.

***Step 9: Balance work with rest and recovery.***   Coach Vince Lombardi said, "Fatigue makes cowards of us all." Overtraining is a major cause of attitude decline as players first physically and then mentally and emotionally burn out. Clever coaches know there is a time for players to switch on to the hard work of soccer, but there is also a time to switch off and let the body and mind recover. An understanding of the need for this balance differentiates between those coaches who can manage a game and those who can manage a season. The latter understand the importance of a winning attitude, and that attitude and energy go together.

***Step 10: Build a PMA club.***   Put all these suggestions together, and we have a soccer club that promotes **P**ositive **M**ental **A**ttitudes. Although positive psychology emphasizes optimism, affirmation, and responsibility, it also stresses a realistic but optimistic interpretation of setbacks. Coaches who can deal with these issues create a motivational environment and surround their players with reasons to succeed rather than reasons to fail. Also, coaches should remember that soccer should be fun—the pleasure always defeating the pressure—and that humor loosens up players physically and mentally and helps create a winning attitude of relaxed readiness.

Table 1.4 offers coaches a chance to assess the extent to which they encourage positive winning attitudes in their players. Coaches must honestly self-assess and determine an action plan for any questions whose answers are not "always." To ensure meaningful appraisal, members of

| TABLE 1.4—Supporting the Psychology of the Player: 20 Key Questions for a Coach | Always | Occasionally | Rarely | Action |
|---|---|---|---|---|
| **1.** Am I positive? | | | | |
| **2.** Am I available? | | | | |
| **3.** Am I fun to be with? | | | | |
| **4.** Do I care for my players? | | | | |
| **5.** Do I know my players as people? | | | | |
| **6.** Do I communicate well? | | | | |
| **7.** Do I listen well? | | | | |
| **8.** Am I honest with my players? | | | | |
| **9.** Am I patient with my players? | | | | |
| **10.** Do I understand player ego? | | | | |
| **11.** Can I manage player mood? | | | | |
| **12.** Do I offer inspiration? | | | | |
| **13.** Am I loyal to my players? | | | | |
| **14.** Do I give clear directions? | | | | |
| **15.** Do I forgive mistakes and move on? | | | | |
| **16.** Do I trust my players? | | | | |
| **17.** Do I offer useful feedback? | | | | |
| **18.** Am I emotionally stable? | | | | |
| **19.** Do I celebrate my players' success? | | | | |
| **20.** Do I offer constant, unwavering support? | | | | |

From B. Beswick, 2010, *Focused for Soccer, Second Edition* (Champaign, IL: Human Kinetics).

coaching teams might answer for each other. In some cases, coaches might ask senior players to complete this; in this case, they must consider any selection of "rarely" and "occasionally" as a cause for concern. The key, then, is translating information into action that demonstrates greater support for the psychological needs of the players.

# Summary

All players and coaches recognize the power of attitude in achieving high levels of performance. The very best players possess both talent and attitude, and even those players a little short on talent can still succeed if they make up for it with a strong and positive attitude.

Attitude is defined here as the translation of thoughts and feelings into action, and coaches judge players' attitudes by their behavior on and off the field. Each player's attitude is shaped by his unique personality, the influence of the people closest to him, and the coaching and playing environment of his soccer club. For female players, attitudes toward soccer begin with social cohesion and the feeling of being needed and cared for within the team, and then move on to task cohesion—being able to function as a team.

Thus performance follows attitude, and attitude is a daily choice made by players. The challenge of soccer is best represented as a battle between positives (feeling fit, playing well, on the team) and negatives (injured, not playing well, not selected). Players and coaches must work together to create positive, winning mind-sets that emphasize the positives and find ways to deal with the negatives.

The personality, style, and skill of the coach have a major impact on the players, and it is often said that coaches get the players they deserve. Coaches must be aware that overtraining, with the resultant fatigue, and overcoaching, with the resultant confusion, can destroy even the most positive team. Similarly, coaches must teach their players to deal with the pressures of success, the expectations of others, and the consequences of failure.

This chapter stresses that a key part of a coach's job is to both understand and shape player attitudes and recognize and deal with negative attitudes. This is the day-to-day challenge for every coach at every level. However, when the battle is won and the team develops good habits, the power of attitude will inevitably lead to greater success in match situations.

# CHAPTER 2

# Player Attitude: Assessment and Profiling

The mind is the athlete, the body simply the means it uses to run faster, hit further, or box better.

**Bryce Courtenay, South African author**

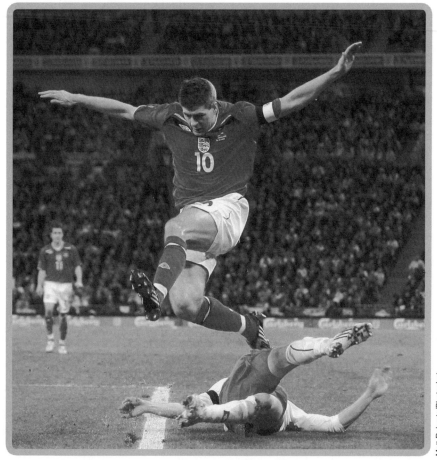

Matt Roberts/Photoshot

t was clear that, even as a young player, the Liverpool midfield player Steven Gerrard had enormous talent but there were doubts about his attitude. Steven was fiercely competitive but lacked control, often getting injured or sent off after unwise tackles. Fortunately his coach, Steve Heighway, sought help, and Steven slowly brought his competitive fire under control. Now Steven has both talent and a disciplined attitude and would be considered a complete player.

Not all players compete with the intensity Gerrard produces every week. Some commit physically but do not engage mentally and are sometimes known as "headless chickens." Others show physical and mental engagement but lack the passion to win. The player all coaches seek engages physically, mentally, and emotionally.

The aim of every soccer player, and the coaches guiding them, should be to develop both the necessary talent and attitude to be considered a complete player. Table 2.1 lists some of the demands soccer players will face. Players can mark in the appropriate columns whether they think the demands are mental, physical, or both. There are no right or wrong answers. Table 2.1 is not an assessment but an exercise. Players may surprise themselves by concluding that much of the challenge of soccer is mental.

### TABLE 2.1—Demands of Soccer

Read the list of key demands in the left-hand column and then check the appropriate columns indicating whether you think the demand is a mental or physical challenge—or both.

| Demand | Physical | Mental | Both |
|---|---|---|---|
| Ability to work hard | | | |
| Endurance and explosive energy | | | |
| Commitment to keep learning | | | |
| Competitiveness | | | |
| Ability to overcome fear of injury | | | |
| Willingness to take responsibility | | | |
| Ability to concentrate | | | |
| Composure in the heat of battle | | | |
| Willingness to sacrifice for the team | | | |
| Willingness to withstand criticism | | | |
| Ability to cope with success or failure | | | |
| High level of tactical awareness | | | |
| Intelligence to make good decisions | | | |

From B. Beswick, 2010, *Focused for Soccer, Second Edition* (Champaign, IL: Human Kinetics).

# The Perfect Player

One of the tasks I like to ask coaches to do is to visualize and describe the perfect game, working from the end backward. The better coaches will quickly and easily outline the physical, technical, and tactical aspects they consider essential. The best coaches, often with considerable and hard-fought experience behind them, will extend their description to include the concept of a winning attitude. They have witnessed perfect games in which the difference in the unfolding contest has been the superior mental and emotional preparation of the winning team.

When I conduct coaches' workshops I often ask this question: "What wins soccer games?" In general, the response always stresses the importance of a winning attitude.

| | |
|---|---|
| Winning attitude | (50%) |
| Defensive organization | (10%) |
| Attacking organization | (10%) |
| Transition organization | (10%) |
| Set plays (for instance, free kicks) | (10%) |
| Special players | (5%) |
| Luck (such as referees' calls) | (5%) |

When I ask players to describe their best performance, I am far more likely to hear about thoughts and feelings. Players often recall how they overcame anxiety and experienced a surge of confidence that fueled an unprecedented performance. Both coaches and players emphasize the importance of getting the right attitude to winning a game.

Although no player is perfect, it is useful for players and coaches to consider the end point of their work and ask this question: "How would a perfect player react to the many challenging situations that can occur on the soccer field?" Miller (1997) reports on just such an exercise conducted by the English men's and women's hockey teams preparing for the Olympic Games. The players worked through hypothetical situations in groups and decided how the perfect player would react. This led to a general agreement about what was and was not acceptable behavior for dealing with these situations, and what standard the players would use to assess themselves. Miller found this exercise developed team understanding and cohesiveness—and contributed to improved performance.

Table 2.2 adapts this exercise for soccer players and illustrates that the perfect player possesses mental and emotional skills to match physical and technical skills. There are no correct answers, but responses from players could bring about an excellent team discussion with the coaches.

| TABLE 2.2—The Perfect Soccer Player | |
|---|---|
| **Situation** | **The perfect player responds by . . .** |
| Inconsistent refereeing | |
| Unfair criticism | |
| Coming on as a substitute | |
| Recovery from injury | |
| A run of defeats | |
| Making mistakes | |
| Mistakes by teammates | |
| Crowd pressure | |
| Receiving a yellow card | |
| Being substituted in a game | |
| Being a goal down | |
| Being a goal up | |
| The big game challenge | |
| Dips in form | |
| Intimidation by opponents | |

From B. Beswick, 2010, *Focused for Soccer, Second Edition* (Champaign, IL: Human Kinetics).

# Understanding the Complete Player

To help coaches and players appreciate the need to place attitude training at the heart of their work, I have created a complete player profile. This emphasizes that players and their performances should be analyzed and assessed against six criteria. Figure 2.1 (page 28) illustrates the complete player profile, describing physical, technical, and tactical criteria as the "hardware" of the player, and mental, emotional, and lifestyle criteria as the "software." It illustrates in broad terms the foundation of the work coaches must carry out in developing players. A well-thought-out training program for players must

- present the players with a *physical challenge,*
- develop *technique* by repetition,
- ensure *tactical* preparation,
- highlight the *mental training* taking place,
- test *emotional* self-control under pressure, and
- reflect *lifestyle* preparation and readiness to commit to soccer.

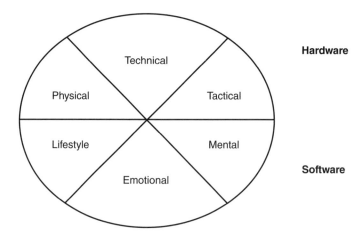

FIGURE 2.1   Complete player profile.

These are the developmental steps coaches and players should work on in order to move toward a more complete performance. However, the following points should be noted:

■ Complete performance is multifaceted; the player is dependent on all facets functioning together.

■ Complete performance is relative to the age and gender of the player. It is vital that youth coaches understand the development patterns of young boys or girls so that they appreciate, for example, the youngster who develops early or late, either physically or emotionally.

■ Complete performance is continually evolving. Ajax in Holland, one of the most famous soccer clubs in the world, rated young players with a system based on the acronym TIPS, which they used to evaluate technique, intelligence, personality, and speed. At a coaches' conference, the head coach for youth revealed that at 8 years of age, speed and technique accounted for 80 percent of the basis for selection. At 18 years of age, however, the intelligence and personality of the player accounted for 80 percent of the basis for selection. The profile of the complete player is continually evolving.

■ Performance problems can originate from any area. Players and coaches must look beyond physical and technical evaluation to assess underlying mental, emotional, and even lifestyle issues. Coaches must see the person as well as the performer and spot those early signs that indicate potential barriers to performance.

■ If coaches or players feel unable to undertake this analysis themselves, they should seek the help of experts. Players and coaches increasingly talk to sport scientists, and they may find themselves the center of a multiskilled support team, as illustrated in the example shown in figure 2.2.

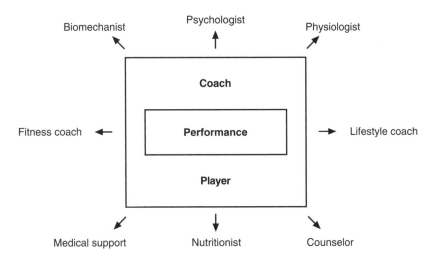

FIGURE 2.2  Players and coaches are at the center of a multiskilled support team.

■ Players will never have perfect profiles, so they must work with the coach and support team to recognize their unique style and learn to manage it to the best effect—playing to their strengths and containing their weaknesses.

■ The pursuit of complete performance will always be affected by the player's particular situation. When I have exhausted all methods to make a player happy and successful, I have to conclude that the player should seek a new club. Often the change itself can stimulate progress. When Jim Smith, the former manager of Derby County in the English Premier League, had difficulty with a couple of players who resisted change, I quoted some Ernest Hemingway to him. "The dogs bark, but the caravan moves on." Jim got the message, a couple of players moved on, and we continued to introduce change to the club.

# Player Assessment— Strengths and Weaknesses

Before a player plans a route to becoming a more complete player, she needs to assess her present strengths and weaknesses. Having identified the priorities for change, the player can collaborate with the coach to establish a series of short- and long-term goals.

The assessment exercises presented here are quick, easy to understand, and acceptable to a soccer culture that can be wary of such tests. The subjective nature of these assessments means that we must take care in interpreting the responses, but I have found a general consistency between the theoretical response and the observed performance.

Such player assessments or profiles offer many benefits:

● Players begin to understand their individual strengths and weaknesses and learn more about themselves.

● Lines of communication are opened up between player and coach.

● Players begin to take more responsibility for their own progress.

● Training objectives can be more clearly established.

● Player and coach can monitor changes from season to season.

● Each player can be benchmarked against the rest of the squad.

● The team can be profiled, and this can influence tactical decisions.

● Recruiting can become more specific as we begin to understand more clearly what we want from our players.

## Assessment by Triangulation

When I joined the staff of the England under-18 soccer team, Howard Wilkinson, head coach at the time, had the problem of selecting a few players from the many available for tryouts. Each player was supported by one recommendation. I suggested that we increase the number of evaluations to three, allowing us to use the process of triangulation.

Triangulation involves asking three respected contacts who would know the player—and at least one who would have directly coached the player—for their opinion. Consistent messages, for or against the player, ensure a more valid assessment of the player's strengths and weaknesses.

## Complete Player Assessments

Because complete performance in soccer is multifaceted, a weakness in one area can lead to an overall performance problem. Table 2.3 asks the players to assess themselves on the six elements of complete performance. Coaches should explain carefully the meaning of each of the six elements and then have the player make an honest self-assessment.

At a coaching conference I asked over 100 coaches to rate player A and player B (the examples in our table 2.3), both of whom at the time were English men's national team players. The average of the responses clearly shows player A to be a complete player but perhaps one who needs to watch a tendency to overreact emotionally. Player B is extremely gifted technically but incomplete holistically. In his case, a poor lifestyle might cause physical, mental, and emotional damage. The superb technical ability of player B subsequently got him to the international level, but his character could not keep him there.

These examples reinforce our message to young players that talent opens the door, but character gets them through to the other side. Talent without character is not talent.

### TABLE 2.3—Complete Player Rating Scale

Assess each aspect of performance on a scale of 1 to 10 using high scores to indicate excellence. Players A and B are examples.

| Aspect of performance | Player A | Player B | Player self-assessment | Coach's rating |
|---|---|---|---|---|
| Physical | 9 | 6 | | |
| Technical | 8 | 10 | | |
| Tactical | 8 | 9 | | |
| Mental | 9 | 6 | | |
| Emotional | 7 | 5 | | |
| Lifestyle | 9 | 4 | | |
| Total | 50 | 40 | | |

From B. Beswick, 2010, *Focused for Soccer, Second Edition* (Champaign, IL: Human Kinetics).

To develop an action plan for improvement, players should assess themselves and compare their rating with that given by the coaches. This is not a foolproof exercise, of course, and players and coaches may alter the weighting of the elements or interpret the responses more specifically according to personality or position played. Be wary also of lifestyle assessments that may be hearsay rather than fact. What is true, though, is that this quick, simple, but reasonably accurate exercise raises awareness, gives early warning signals about particular problem elements of performance, and opens up the discussion on a player's psychology.

Gareth Southgate and his fellow defenders at Middlesbrough enjoyed this exercise to the extent they felt comfortable rating each other and sensibly discussing score differences. They then went on to complete table 2.4 (page 32), identifying their view of key criteria in the profile of a complete defender.

### Assessment by Hardware-Software Rating

Player performance is a combination of physical and mental skills. Players and coaches often want a quick way to determine the relative strengths and weaknesses of these areas. The physical skills are the hardware and the mental skills the software. Performance requires both, and the well-known computer phrase "Garbage in, garbage out" highlights the need for developing a player's mental state. Table 2.5 (page 32) shows the software profile of an international player I had the honor to work with.

Figure 2.3 (page 33) graphs the relationship between a player's hardware and software skills. Coaches are asked to assess each on a level of 1 (poor)

## TABLE 2.4—The Complete Defender

| Performance areas | Key qualities |
|---|---|
| Physical | 1. Strength and power<br>2. Pace and sharpness<br>3. Endurance and fitness<br>4. Agility and balance<br>5. Presence |
| Technical | 1. Positional sense—ballside or blindside<br>2. Body position<br>3. Tackling and heading skills<br>4. Ball control<br>5. Distribution |
| Tactical | 1. Ability to read the game (states and stages)<br>2. Understanding team shape and game plan<br>3. Knowing your job<br>4. Anticipation—reading situations early<br>5. Communication and leadership |
| Mental | 1. Mental toughness and positivity<br>2. Concentration (90+ minutes)<br>3. Self-belief and confidence<br>4. Responsibility<br>5. Courage on and off the ball |
| Emotional | 1. Passion—about defending well<br>2. Composure or coolness under fire<br>3. Ability to recover from mistakes and move on<br>4. Supportive of your teammates and team first<br>5. Enjoyment of your job, make defending fun |
| Lifestyle | 1. Sacrifice, dedication, and professionalism<br>2. Balance of work, rest, recovery, and home life<br>3. Diet—healthy eating<br>4. Surrounding yourself with good people<br>5. Being a good person as well as good player |

## TABLE 2.5—Software Profile of a Male International Player

| Performance areas | Key qualities |
|---|---|
| **Mental** | 1. Needs every game or training session to be serious<br>2. Does not see problems, only challenges<br>3. Wants coaches to challenge, not respect, him<br>4. Independent, proud, needs recognition<br>5. Frustrated when limited by team or coaches |
| **Emotional** | 1. Gets upset by poor standards—players or coaches<br>2. Good emotional intelligence and fine leader<br>3. Excellent emotional control during games<br>4. Upset by mistakes but recovers well<br>5. Defeats hurt—needs help postgame |
| **Lifestyle** | 1. Very low-maintenance player<br>2. Staying fit is way of life for him<br>3. Understands and accepts sacrifice<br>4. Demands the same standards from teammates<br>5. Excellent role model and captain |

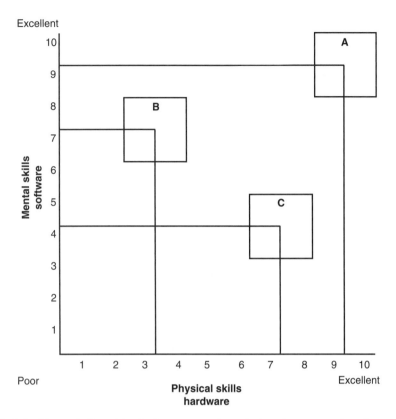

FIGURE 2.3  The relationship between a player's hardware and software skills. Player A is a complete player with no significant weaknesses; player B is mentally strong with possible physical weaknesses; and player C is physically strong but may have mental weaknesses.

to 10 (excellent). Clearly, this is a quick and rough guide, but informed assessors can provide a quick and useful profile on which to base future work with individual players. If a coach were to map all his players on the graph, he would have an immediate picture of the team profile—for example, a team high on hardware, low on software.

Recently I had a chance to ask Phil Neville, captain of Everton Football Club in the English Premier League, how he would rate himself. Phil was quite clear he was in the B category when it came to physical skills, and his great career had been driven by excellent software skills.

## Profile of Winning Attitudes

After reviewing many soccer case studies, I put together 24 key statements that form a profile of the mental and emotional skills of a player with a winning attitude. These are listed in table 2.6 (page 34), and players are asked to rate themselves for each statement.

The scores have a range of 24 to 120, and clearly the higher the score, the more the player can be considered mentally strong. Scores below 72

## TABLE 2.6—Winning Attitudes: A Self-Rating Questionnaire

Here are some statements that coaches and players can use to describe the psychological qualities needed for excellence. Rate yourself for each statement using a scale of 1 to 5. A 5 indicates the statement is definitely true of you, and a 1 indicates it is absolutely not true of you. Scores between 1 and 5 would reflect partial truths. The total score is useful only when compared within the group or to a coach's assessment; this questionnaire is more useful for increasing self-awareness and developing an action plan to deal with weaknesses.

| Statement: Circle appropriate number. | False | | | | True |
|---|---|---|---|---|---|
| **1.** I am always confident in my abilities. | 1 | 2 | 3 | 4 | 5 |
| **2.** Challenge is fun. | 1 | 2 | 3 | 4 | 5 |
| **3.** I always see myself performing at my best. | 1 | 2 | 3 | 4 | 5 |
| **4.** I keep highs and lows in equal perspective. | 1 | 2 | 3 | 4 | 5 |
| **5.** You can rely on me to stay self-disciplined. | 1 | 2 | 3 | 4 | 5 |
| **6.** I am willing to sacrifice to achieve. | 1 | 2 | 3 | 4 | 5 |
| **7.** I enjoy every practice and game. | 1 | 2 | 3 | 4 | 5 |
| **8.** I am always cool under pressure. | 1 | 2 | 3 | 4 | 5 |
| **9.** I feel good about myself as a player. | 1 | 2 | 3 | 4 | 5 |
| **10.** I know my strengths and weaknesses. | 1 | 2 | 3 | 4 | 5 |
| **11.** I recover from mistakes well. | 1 | 2 | 3 | 4 | 5 |
| **12.** Distractions never affect my game. | 1 | 2 | 3 | 4 | 5 |
| **13.** I am willing to work as hard as it takes. | 1 | 2 | 3 | 4 | 5 |
| **14.** I will take risks when the situation is right. | 1 | 2 | 3 | 4 | 5 |
| **15.** I practice proper relaxation and recovery methods. | 1 | 2 | 3 | 4 | 5 |
| **16.** I respond well to useful criticism. | 1 | 2 | 3 | 4 | 5 |
| **17.** I push harder even when it hurts. | 1 | 2 | 3 | 4 | 5 |
| **18.** I enjoy being part of a team effort. | 1 | 2 | 3 | 4 | 5 |
| **19.** I never allow negative thinking in games. | 1 | 2 | 3 | 4 | 5 |
| **20.** Practicing with intensity is important to me. | 1 | 2 | 3 | 4 | 5 |
| **21.** I recover well from setbacks in games. | 1 | 2 | 3 | 4 | 5 |
| **22.** I will persist until I achieve. | 1 | 2 | 3 | 4 | 5 |
| **23.** I always take responsibility for my actions. | 1 | 2 | 3 | 4 | 5 |
| **24.** I need to be the best I can be. | 1 | 2 | 3 | 4 | 5 |

| Scoring box | Player total | Coach's total | Team average |
|---|---|---|---|
| All questions | | | |
| Self-concept 3, 4, 9, 10, 15, 16, 18, 19 | | | |
| Motivation 1, 6, 7, 13, 17, 20, 22, 24 | | | |
| Mental toughness 2, 5, 8, 11, 12, 14, 21, 23 | | | |

From B. Beswick, 2010, *Focused for Soccer, Second Edition* (Champaign, IL: Human Kinetics).

would generally indicate a player with attitude problems, and coaches should undertake a closer analysis of particular low-scoring questions. This should provide the beginnings of an action plan to help the player develop mental strength (see table 2.7 as an example).

However, coaches can go a step further in profiling because the statements are organized to reflect three key psychological areas—self-concept, motivation, and mental toughness. The scoring box at the end of table 2.6 can be used to tally the various scores.

By separating the scores for these three sets of questions, players or coaches can more specifically identify some general trends of strengths and weaknesses. Naturally, some of the most interesting talking points are the differences of opinion between the players' rating of themselves and their rating by the coaches.

## TABLE 2.7—Winning Attitudes: Individual Profile

Player's name: Lee Carsley

| Psychological focus | Player score (max. 40) | Psychologist's comments |
|---|---|---|
| Self-concept: The way you view and value yourself as a player | 23 | To your credit you recognize the problem and give yourself the lowest score of the squad. The coaches feel this is holding you back, and you must become more positive about yourself. |
| Motivation: Your willingness to pay the price | 35 | A good score that reflects your desire to do well. The coaches also praise your commitment and pride in performance. |
| Mental toughness: The strength of your focus, the durability of your concentration | 31 | There is concern about your ability to handle pressure with emotional control. In the position you play, you must combine passion with discipline and composure. |

**Player action plan: The key is belief in yourself.**

**1.** You have to be more positive about yourself and surround yourself with positive influences.

**2.** Set yourself small, achievable targets for this season to improve your confidence and, just as important, the confidence of others in you (look good, feel good, play good).

**3.** Practices, and your attitude to them, are very important in changing attitudes toward you.

**4.** When you make errors or lose control emotionally, try to remember the causes and create a plan not to let them happen again.

**5.** Don't get depressed—you have achieved a great deal so far, and much of what is wrong here can only be changed by experience.

**6.** When you get forward on runs, you have to express commitment and the conviction you can (a) get into the box, and (b) score. Set targets for yourself.

**7.** Be patient and take the long-term view of your career.

In chapter 1, we looked at how Lee Carsley got the message about mental and emotional development. Lee's rapid and exciting progress began after he completed the winning attitudes questionnaire and began to discuss with me how to improve his low self-concept and poor emotional control. A compelling demonstration of the improvement in Lee's self-concept is that he agreed to share his first results, table 2.7, with you.

## Performance Problems

As we have established, performance problems can be physical, technical, tactical, mental, emotional, or perhaps the result of a poor lifestyle. In the past, players and coaches examined only physical, technical, and tactical issues in relation to performance problems, but we are now becoming more aware of the potential impact of mental, emotional, and lifestyle issues. One note of caution is that the player and coach must be sure that a biological or medical condition is not the cause of the behavior weakness. An important part of my work is to review players' physical condition with the team doctor before I concentrate on potential mental and emotional factors. The Rory Delap case study illustrates the need to be cautious in the diagnostic stage.

In observing players, it is important that I help the coaches by identifying reasons other than the physical or technical that might be adversely

### Rory Delap Gives Us Food for Thought

The case of Rory Delap, when he was a young player at Derby County, illustrates that performance problems can be multifaceted, and that coaches should be wary of making quick judgments.

Rory plays wingback, a position that makes great physical demands on the player, requiring both endurance and explosive energy. After an excellent start to the season, Rory suddenly lost form, especially in the second half of games when the frequency and length of his supporting runs would diminish.

While the coaches privately discussed Rory's loss of confidence, lack of ability, inability to understand tactics, and a host of other potential reasons, I approached Rory and asked him his views. What emerged was a problem of nutrition, easy to understand and easy to cure. Rory had recently left the club's hotel to live in his first purchased house, and he couldn't cook! As his nutritional intake plunged, so did his performance. He was running on empty! A series of arrangements, including a telephone call to his mother, were put in place, and the problem resolved itself. Rory became an outstanding player at Stoke City.

affecting a player's performance. To do this, I need to observe players at practice and in games, when I may be the only spectator not watching the ball. Most important is that I build relationships with players so they can feel comfortable in sharing problems with me.

Performance problems can often cause an emotional overreaction. Players and coaches must be careful not to jump to conclusions. Employing a series of questions might help identify the true cause of the problem:

> Q1. Is this a "can't do" or a "won't do"? If the former, the problem is clearly technical; if the latter, it's one of attitude.
>
> Q2. When and how do problems occur?
>
> Q3. Are problems restricted to one element of performance, or do they affect several areas of play?
>
> Q4. What thoughts and feelings does the player associate with the problem?
>
> Q5. Are problems the result of pressure? Is the player OK in practice but not in the game?

Combining the answers to these questions with the follow-up questions in table 2.8, players and coaches can be more objective and can more accurately and quickly identify the causes of performance problems.

If "can't do" is the answer, then the problem is a recruitment or training issue. The action plan might be extra specific work on the training ground. If "won't do" is the issue, then clearly it is a motivation or attitude problem, and the action plan might involve discussion, counseling, or the use of a sport psychologist.

### TABLE 2.8—Understanding a Performance Problem

| Starter question | Follow-up questions | Yes (✓) | No (X) | Maybe (?) |
|---|---|---|---|---|
| Is this a "can't do" problem? | • Is this a physical problem?<br>• Is this a technical problem?<br>• Is this a tactical problem? | | | |
| Is this a "won't do" problem? | • Is this a mental problem?<br>• Is this an emotional problem?<br>• Is this a lifestyle problem? | | | |
| Conclusion: | | | | |
| Action: | | | | |

From B. Beswick, 2010, *Focused for Soccer, Second Edition* (Champaign, IL: Human Kinetics).

Of course, to understand performance problems, you have to understand performance. I constantly urge young sport psychologists to work on understanding the game and what players and coaches are trying to achieve. I once sent a rather naive student to observe a local semiprofessional club. After the game, the coach asked for his input. The student immediately criticized the coach for not removing number 10 at halftime.

"Why?" asked the coach.

"He touched the ball only five times," said the student.

"But he scored twice," said the coach as he ended the conversation.

In my follow-up with the student, I gave him the example of Michael Owen's performance when England beat Germany 5-1. Michael had only 75 seconds in total possession of the ball but he scored three goals. Michael's performance strength was not his physical involvement in the game but rather his mental and emotional control, which allowed him to seize the moments and define the game.

## Creating Self-Managing Players

An important by-product of engaging in assessment exercises is that players begin to think about their performance and take ownership of both physical and mental development. One of the benefits of having a sport psychologist working with a soccer club is that players will become more involved in their own performance:

**1.** Players will be asked to self-reference—to judge their own performances, to evaluate their strengths and weaknesses, and to come to terms with their attitudes and feelings rather than simply listening to the coach or parent telling them how they should think. As was mentioned in chapter 1, the hardest questions are the ones that players ask themselves.

**2.** Players will engage in self-reflection. Aided by film analysis and the comments of the coaches, and guided by the sport psychologist, players will reflect on their last performance and answer questions such as these:

- What happened?
- What was I thinking and feeling at the time?
- What was good (or bad) about the experience?
- What else could I have done?
- If it happened again, what would I do?
- If I wanted to change this behavior, could I?

We know already that the battle to attain excellent mental and emotional skills is mainly internal—you versus you. These exercises force players to confront themselves and accept responsibility for any progress or change. Using this process builds a high level of intrinsic motivation. Players want to achieve progress for themselves rather than rely on the urgings of a coach or parent, marking an important stage on the way to mental toughness.

This process is especially important to goalkeepers and strikers who are the players most vulnerable to mental and emotional stress. The goalkeeper cannot hide on the soccer field—the keeper either saves the shot or doesn't. Even if it's not the keeper's fault, she will have to pick up the ball from the back of the net. Similarly, all can clearly see that the striker either scores or misses with the chances she is given. For these players, self-referencing and self-reflection are important methods of coping with stress.

## Developing an Action Plan— A Guide for Players

Your action plan to become a more complete player began when you picked up this book. It now continues as you use these quick, easy measures to assess mental and emotional strengths and weaknesses.

You should understand that psychological skills are not magic. It isn't true that some people have them and some don't. Anyone can learn psychological skills at any time and in most places, but like physical skills, effective learning requires good early instruction, repetition, and perseverance. The goal of this book is to raise your awareness of the essential importance of mental and emotional skills in your performance and then to provide you with that good early instruction.

As you proceed through the book you will find many suggestions for improving your mental strength. I suggest that you adopt the following routine in incorporating these ideas into your training and performance philosophy:

- Assess. Use the tools offered to determine your weaknesses.
- Set goals. Decide what you would like to achieve and identify a progressive series of small and relatively easily achieved steps that will take you there. (To help players, I usually ask them to focus on three things they can do well to help their team, plus how they can be a really good team member.)
- Visualize. See yourself as you want to be and check what it will feel like. Use quiet moments with the team such as when traveling on the bus.
- Practice. Act out your visualization and implement it. Decide that "if that happens, then I will respond by such a behavior." Forgive yourself for your mistakes. As with all learning, you will use a trial-and-error pattern. Learning to recover is itself an important skill. Players should commit to practicing mental skills in all aspects of their lives.

For example, they can practice composure and arousal-frustration control just as easily in a traffic jam as at training.

- Monitor. Constantly check your progress, and listen to the comments of those around you. Are they seeing a change? Watch film of yourself in action and reflect on your performance.
- Automate. A relevant saying is "habits save you in big games." Repeat and repeat until you have a new and positive habit.
- Enjoy. Your new behavior will boost your confidence. Reward yourself by enjoying your status as a more complete player.

To help you understand and become familiar with this process, examine the many case studies in this book and check them against this system for developing mental skills.

## Integrating Physical and Mental Skill Development

The message is that the journey to soccer excellence—as both an individual and a team player—must involve training to meet the mental demands of the game as well as the physical and technical demands. Because mind and body must act in unison to meet many of the demands of soccer, this book advocates an approach to learning soccer that combines and reinforces the mind–body link. If physical practice is meant to re-create game conditions, then a thoughtful coach will mention the mental and emotional factors that might well accompany that situation. After all, what would be the point of practicing penalties as a physical exercise only?

Although in some situations, players can practice mental skills in isolation, there are clear benefits when the mind and body link can be positively reinforced in practice and competition. Jim Reardon expressed the view of the sport psychology team responsible for the U.S. track and field team.

> Specifically, we believe that psychological skills training is most effective when it is interwoven into the physical training regimen on a continual basis. The failure to incorporate these skills/abilities into training opens the athlete up to a variety of disruptions in performance. How many times have you seen athletes who were physically prepared struggle through competitions self-consciously burdened by worry and doubt? (1992, conference presentation)

To prevent inadequate mental preparation from undermining excellent physical preparation, coaches should integrate mental skills training into physical routines whenever possible. Figure 2.4 illustrates a model practice designed to achieve this. If, for example, the drill was a 3v1 "keep ball" practice, the coach, besides reinforcing players' technical skills,

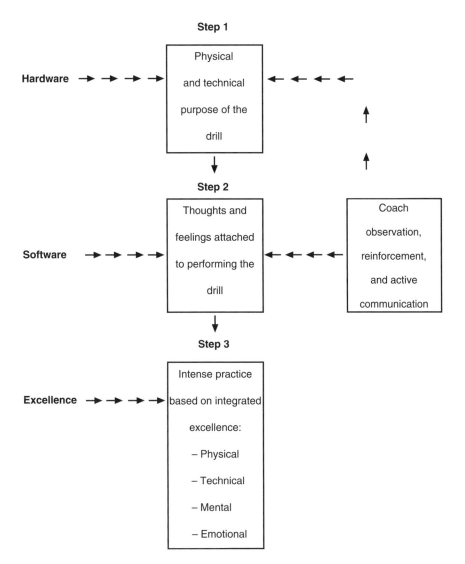

FIGURE 2.4 A model practice integrating physical and mental aspects of performance.

could use the opportunity to program relevant software messages such as concentration on and off the ball, composure (control the defender), challenge (accept the challenge), communication, managing mistakes, and maintaining determination to succeed. All are essential aspects of the successful, complete performance.

Another excellent example was devised by Anson Dorrance, coach of the highly successful women's soccer team at the University of North Carolina. The strategy was simple: Get great players and add psychological strength. To achieve this, the coaches integrated a mental training program with a vigorous physical program. They assessed each drill for the extent to which it would develop mental strength as well as build physical capacity. This produced an intense and exacting practice schedule in which focus, intensity, desire, competitiveness, and mental toughness were essential to survival and success. Here, the muscles were the slaves of the brain.

Such integration, plus the policy of always playing the toughest opponents possible, made the women players of North Carolina confident, highly competitive, and able to cope with the stresses of the big game. The coaches clearly demonstrated a commitment to enhancing the mental and emotional functioning of the players and built this into every aspect of their training and competition.

# Summary

The demands of soccer challenge each player physically, technically, tactically, mentally, emotionally, and in terms of a supportive lifestyle. To reach the highest level, players have to work to improve all these dimensions of performance. This chapter highlights the importance of the attitude or software of the player—mental, emotional, and lifestyle aspects. The aim of every soccer player should be to develop a healthy lifestyle and well-shaped mental and emotional attitudes that allow them to maximize physical, technical, and tactical potential.

In my experience there are very few players who could consider themselves complete players—strong on all dimensions; most have a profile of strengths and weaknesses. It is of great benefit to both coaches and players to use assessment exercises in order to raise awareness of both strengths and weaknesses. Such assessments quickly build up a player performance profile, pinpoint likely performance problems, and stimulate both coach and player to devise an action plan for improvement.

Advice is given on structuring an action plan for improvement where the performance problems are psychological, and the case of Lee Carsley is evidence that early assessment and the right action plan can lead to dramatic psychological improvement. It is emphasized throughout this whole process that the player who wishes to succeed must take responsibility for his own performance and improvement.

Finally, coaches are urged to integrate the improvement of mental strength as a part of the normal physical, technical, and tactical development of players. Attitude training does not necessarily take place in the classroom but rather while dealing with the day-to-day challenge of practicing and playing excellently.

# CHAPTER 3

# Confidence: Building Self-Belief in Players and Teams

Confidence is a bridge connecting expectations
and performance, investment and results.

**R.M. Kanter (2004)**

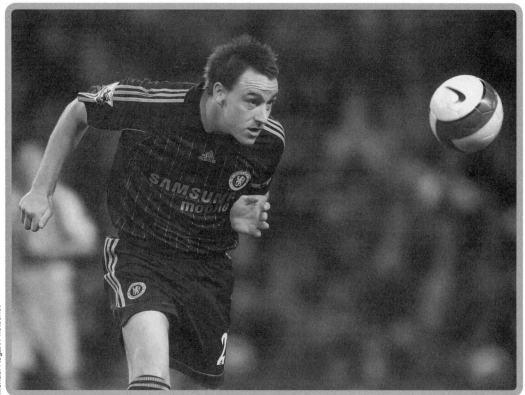

Success in soccer is based on a foundation of player and team confidence—the constant belief that challenges can be overcome. I was honored to be the first team psychologist for the England National Team but met a squad that had clearly lost some confidence. Our first get-together was only a few weeks after the team returned from the World Cup—suffering the usual disappointment from the nation and the predictable media criticism.

Our first objective was to make these very talented young players remember that playing for England is very special. We created a series of short presentations, backed by motivational films, which we titled *The Prize Is Worthwhile*. These were the key messages:

- You can only win the European Nations Cup with England.
- You can only win the World Cup with England.
- You are capable of achieving these dreams.
- The first step is believing and thinking positively.
- We can manage the high expectations placed on us.
- We can deal with the negative consequences of setbacks.
- The captain will be our leader.

With the use of increased communication, the motivational film, and shared ownership of the problem, we slowly rebuilt desire, belief, and the necessary confidence and commitment to set out on a very challenging journey.

The more I work alongside junior, senior, and international players, the more clearly I see that soccer constantly assaults players' confidence. I have come to understand that confidence lies at the heart of successful performance. With confidence, a player will cross the white line and face up to the many demands of competitive soccer. Without confidence, the same player will at some stage withdraw back into a personal and much safer comfort zone.

The central purpose of my work is to help players, coaches, and teams achieve a state of confidence that can stimulate consistently high performance levels and withstand the inevitable setbacks. Figure 3.1 shows the range of confidence-threatening situations any player may face and represents the agenda that coaches and psychologists face in teaching their players the coping skills to deal with the challenge of soccer. All players face these pressures—the successful players are the ones who deal with them and still focus on performing well.

## Confidence Is a Choice

The journey to becoming a more complete player begins by building confidence and then learning to maintain it after setbacks. When players or coaches describe themselves as under pressure, they are really identify-

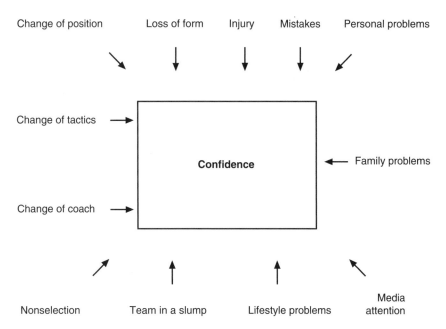

**FIGURE 3.1** Situations that threaten the confidence of both players and coaches.

ing a lack of confidence in dealing with a situation. With confidence, we expect success. Learning something new, like building the mental game plan described in this book, becomes a challenge rather than a problem.

Confidence, though, is a choice; you have to choose to become confident. When I talk to younger players, I illustrate this point by describing (and acting out!) the behavior of two parrots, one perched on each shoulder. One of them is the positive parrot, constantly urging the player to face up to the challenge, saying, "You can do it." The other is the negative parrot, incessantly warning the player, "You can't do it." Clearly, you choose which parrot you listen to.

Once you have made the choice, and it may be a decision faced many times, you must take responsibility for your actions. Successful players build their confidence by concentrating on their contribution to team performance. Rather than blame someone or something else when setbacks happen—a sign of insecurity—they take responsibility and see setbacks as part of a learning curve, not a disaster that could damage confidence.

## Characteristics of Confidence

One of the keys to managing a successful team is the ability to make judgments about a player's ability to cope with the demands of competition. Judging physical readiness is easier than judging mental readiness, so coaches will look for clear messages, both verbal and nonverbal, that the player is confident in her ability to succeed at this level.

Players high in confidence offer such messages by

- having high self-belief—a "can do" attitude;
- projecting a positive image—always displaying confident body language;
- enjoying competition and smiling;
- not worrying unduly about failure or consequences;
- being self-dependent, not seeking to blame others;
- staying calm and collected, showing good self-control;
- talking to themselves and others in an encouraging, positive way;
- concentrating well, both in training and in matches;
- having no need to impress others; and
- accepting themselves while understanding their strengths and weaknesses.

Players low in confidence

- find evidence they are no good,
- worry about what others think about them,
- are very negative—saying "I can't . . . ,"
- have poor concentration (distracted by focusing on what they can't do),
- project a negative image (poor body language),
- become very emotional and think irrationally,
- don't enjoy their sport,
- become dependent on others,
- are blind to any success, and
- focus on failure and worry about the consequences.

All these characteristics reflect a player's level of confidence in her ability to cope with the challenge of soccer. Confident thinking initiates a chain reaction that provides a high level of energy—the fuel of positive performance. Table 3.1 shows the relationship between confidence and positive energy, illustrating that a confident state of mind leads to positive emotions, high energy, and successful performance.

One of the ways I help coaches is by using my freedom from specific responsibility in practice to observe players and check their body language, comments, and performance for clues to their general level of confidence. I once remarked to coach Steve McClaren after practice that I felt that Derby's Italian star, Stefano Eranio, was a little down. The coach called him at home that evening, the player was delighted, and a two-hour conversation put Eranio's world right.

| TABLE 3.1—Relationship Between Confidence and Energy | | |
|---|---|---|
| | **Player A** | **Player B** |
| Attitude ↓ | Confident | Lacking confidence |
| Emotions ↓ | Excited, vigorous | Anxious, frustrated |
| Energy ↓ | Positive | Negative |
| Potential performance | Successful | Unsuccessful |

# Steps to Building Confidence

Although the building of confidence is an ongoing task, players should consider certain key steps to find what works for them.

## Stay in the Game

When Jackie Stewart, the famous Scottish racing driver, allowed the television cameras into his home, viewers quickly noticed that he had retained only one trophy from the many he had won. Jackie explained that he had won that trophy in a race that had taught him an invaluable lesson early in his career. He had been lying in seventh position with six laps to go, had given up hope, and was cruising. By the end of the race, all six of the cars in front had withdrawn with mistakes or problems. Jackie had learned that by staying in the game and competing as long and as hard as he could, he might make his own luck.

Confidence is built on experience, with the greatest boost going to the player with the knowledge that he recognizes the situation and knows what to expect. Players have to be willing to go through the fire of fears, mistakes, defeats, and criticism to build the foundation of experience they need for confidence at the highest levels.

The next time you watch an Olympic champion celebrate success, remember that many of them failed in their first appearance at the Games. But they had been through the fire, had learned from their mistakes, and had stayed in the game before succeeding at the second or even third attempt. Do you think they feel it was worth it?

## Commit to Good Preparation

Confidence comes from success, and success in soccer is more likely if you run out on the field knowing you have done everything you could to prepare for situations that might bring pressure. Clearly, lack of preparation can result in the stress (absence of confidence) of not being able to handle such pressure. "If you are not preparing to win, you are preparing to fail" is a phrase often quoted. Good coaches take the view that if they have prepared properly, the players will be confident that no surprises will appear on the field of play; the players will be prepared for every eventuality.

For Michael Johnson, the 200- and 400-meter gold medalist in the 1996 Olympic Games, confidence comes from belief in preparation and commitment: "My confidence is knowing that I have probably trained harder than anyone I am going to run against. . . . that translates into the belief that if I am in a race, I am going to win" (1996).

## See the Big Picture

Confidence is based on continual achievement, however small, so it is important to maintain progress in all aspects of soccer development. When a player suffers a loss of confidence, it is often because of the failure of one aspect of his game. Too much attention to this component can obscure the fact that the player is progressing well in other areas. He must be reminded of this!

Thus it is important for players and coaches to keep the big picture in mind when reviewing progress. My role is to help players change their view of things, often from negative to positive, a process I call reframing. Instead of overemphasizing one problem, we create a new picture that includes many aspects of play to be confident about and one area that needs special attention. We can then view this as a challenge, not a problem.

## Build a Tick Stepladder

Most research on goal setting describes the route to high self-esteem and confidence as a tick stepladder in which every achievement, no matter how small, is recorded and rewarded. Lee Carsley had low self-esteem and confidence but agreed to a 21-step change program. Each day I set Lee a different task to achieve: be early, be smart, be first on the field, be last off the field, and so on. As Lee achieved each task—and we gave him a tick (also known as a check)—he built his own stepladder to higher self-esteem and confidence. Achieving small goals regularly, and feeling good about it, is the way to build confidence and coping skills for the big goals.

This approach is useful for players who have suffered a dramatic loss of self-esteem and confidence from loss of form or when facing a long recovery from injury. Martin Taylor, a former Derby County goalkeeper of exceptional courage, faced a two-year recovery from a severe injury. With his wife, he planned every step of his recovery on a large chart on the kitchen wall at home. Every day, every exercise, every hospital visit, and every possible sign of progress was given a tick and recorded. Neither

Martin nor his wife would accept any loss of self-esteem, and both were confident that Martin would soon be back playing professional soccer. He returned far sooner than predicted, with greater mental toughness.

Players and coaches should have dreams and visions but should make their ladder one of small and reasonably attainable steps. Coaches can structure practices and their game schedule to build in early success. This early success will boost confidence and motivate the team to face the more difficult challenges on the way.

Coaches should encourage players to complete table 3.2. Players high on confidence should be scoring a total of 40 or above. Scores below 40 indicate a general lack of confidence. Players must pay special attention to any individual score of 2 or less; these indicate confidence problems that should be discussed with the coach.

| TABLE 3.2—Self-Assessment of Confidence for Players | | | | | | |
|---|---|---|---|---|---|---|
| How confident are you of | | Low | | | High | |
| 1. | making the team? | 1 | 2 | 3 | 4 | 5 |
| 2. | your own abilities? | 1 | 2 | 3 | 4 | 5 |
| 3. | your preparation for games? | 1 | 2 | 3 | 4 | 5 |
| 4. | your fitness to last the game? | 1 | 2 | 3 | 4 | 5 |
| 5. | doing your job tactically? | 1 | 2 | 3 | 4 | 5 |
| 6. | staying self-disciplined? | 1 | 2 | 3 | 4 | 5 |
| 7. | dealing with the distractions? | 1 | 2 | 3 | 4 | 5 |
| 8. | dealing with the unexpected? | 1 | 2 | 3 | 4 | 5 |
| 9. | recovering well from mistakes? | 1 | 2 | 3 | 4 | 5 |
| 10. | handling any criticism? | 1 | 2 | 3 | 4 | 5 |
| | Total score | | | | | |

From B. Beswick, 2010, *Focused for Soccer, Second Edition* (Champaign, IL: Human Kinetics).

## Program the Inner Tape

As we move through each day encountering a stream of varying situations, we constantly talk to ourselves. Our inner tape provides a recording of our state of mind, with those parrots I mentioned helping us determine whether we talk ourselves up or talk ourselves down. Confidence, therefore, is the result of what we say to ourselves about what we think about ourselves.

Players with confidence program their inner tape with positive self-talk, whereas low-confidence players feed their anxiety by using negative self-talk. Because we know (see table 3.1) that performance follows attitude and that attitude is based on the confidence a player feels in a given situation, then every player clearly needs training in using positive self-talk and rejecting negative self-talk.

Table 3.3 shows the results of an exercise in self-talk conducted with the England women's senior team. This team had proved quite anxious and vulnerable to negative self-talk. The exercise, then, was one of opening up the fears and anxieties contained in negative self-talk and then working together to find positive self-talk responses that could replace them.

When I speak to players either individually or as a team, I always try to identify where they are coming from, mentally and emotionally. What doubts, fears, and anxieties are playing on their inner tapes at that moment? Of course, my job is to work with the coaches to help the player or team program the tape with different and positive messages. Even in the worst circumstances, successful players and teams can find a way to be positive. Players should remember this adage: "What happens to you is not nearly as important as how you react to what happens to you."

### TABLE 3.3—Confidence and Self-Talk

Results of an exercise with the England women's senior team: changing negative self-talk into positive self-talk

| Negative self-talk | Positive self-talk |
| --- | --- |
| I'm not willing to go through this. | I am still willing to pay the price. |
| I'm not good enough. | Trust the coaches—they selected me. |
| I won't cope. | I have the experience now to deal with anything. |
| I'm not ready. | I'm as ready as I'll ever be. |
| I'm afraid of criticism. | I'll take responsibility for my game and whatever criticism comes. |
| What about injury? | I always play hard and accept injuries as part of the game. |
| I'll make mistakes. | I may make mistakes, but I know how to recover. |
| What if I miss the shot? | I'll get the next one. |
| What if they score first? | I'll work even harder. |
| I'll have a bad game, and we'll lose. | I worry only about things I can control, so I will play my best and stay in the present. |
| I don't look good. | I love this uniform, and I feel really proud. |
| We aren't tough enough. | I am happy to walk into the valley of the shadow of death because I know my teammates are the meanest bitches in there! |

## Build a Positive Support Group

Although I urge players to take responsibility for building their own self-concept and confidence, every player is influenced, positively or negatively, by the comments received from family and friends, from those who surround them daily. For all players, it is essential that the people they share their feelings with—family, partner, teammates, counselor—reinforce their belief in themselves and their motivation to pursue soccer excellence. Such emotional reinforcement is especially needed by female players, whose decision to play soccer often involves a difficult choice in competition with many other demands on their time and resources. The background influence of fans and the media may also be important.

Parents, for example, can be part of the problem or part of the solution. Players who receive loving and well-balanced support from their parents are far more likely to overcome the challenges of soccer than those who must try to fulfill parental egos and dreams. Dan Marino, the great

### Confidence and the Striker Who Can't Score

I have mentioned before the special case of goalkeepers and strikers. For them, reframing is especially important. When Dean Sturridge, the former Derby County striker, had a spell when he couldn't score goals, his whole game fell apart. After discussion with Steve McClaren, then the Derby County coach, we asked Dean to observe one of his favorite players—striker Ian Wright, then of Arsenal—and record every contribution Ian made to his team's play. After joint discussion, we agreed on five essential elements of a striker's play:

1. Scoring goals
2. Making goals or assists
3. Making forward runs and being available for passes
4. Holding the ball up and bringing teammates into play
5. Pressuring defenders when they have the ball

We then assessed Dean's present performances on each of these five elements on a score of 1 to 10. Clearly, his marks were low on scoring goals, but he was surprised at the positive scores on other aspects of his play.

The smaller view was that he was not scoring goals—the bigger, more helpful picture was that he was contributing to the team in other ways. Of course, strikers must score goals, but they all have barren periods that they must recover from. Dean's case is an example of how to deal positively with such a problem—reframing the picture, maintaining overall confidence, and buying time until the next goal comes along, the occurrence that will provide the ultimate confidence boost.

American football quarterback, was fortunate to have a father who used to leave notes for him saying, "I love you—win or fail."

Handling key relationships is a lifestyle skill of the complete player. Part of my counseling always includes how well my players are dealing with the tricky balance of the demands of soccer and the demands of home. On many occasions, I have been asked to deal with a soccer problem that, upon investigation, turned out to be a problem at home that was spilling over into soccer performance.

Players must be urged to ignore the moaners. Confidence is a choice. On one occasion, I saw a player take a positive action at halftime in a match by suddenly taking all his clothes and moving to another spot in the dressing room. When I later asked him why he did this, he explained that the new player next to him was moaning nonstop. Although the team was down 0-1, the first player felt the game was still theirs to win, and he did not want his confidence affected. Players, coaches, parents, and friends should always remember coach Vince Lombardi's belief: "Confidence is contagious. So is lack of confidence."

## Screen Out Distractions

Later in this book I describe mental toughness as remaining positive in the face of adversity. As figure 3.1 (page 45) has illustrated, soccer undoubtedly provides a range of confidence-threatening situations. Bill Parcells, outstanding American football coach, regards highly the ability of players to ignore things they cannot control while concentrating on the one thing they can control—their minds:

> It's easy to get diverted by all the variables outside your control, to let them eat away at your vision and self-confidence. But details will doom you—lose faith in yourself and you will fulfill your own worst prophecy. (1995, 15)

Successful players and teams discipline their minds to accept only positive and supportive messages; they actively reject negative interference. Clever coaches work hard to create an environment that limits the possibility of negative interference. Teams at home thus have the advantage because they can more easily control their environment and minimize distractions. For instance, for the last 25 years, Anfield Stadium, the home of Liverpool, has had an awesome reputation for undermining the confidence of visiting teams. To meet this challenge, visiting teams must set these objectives for their visit to Anfield:

● Beat the environment—play the game and not the occasion.

● Concentrate on their game and not Liverpool's.

● Focus only on the things that are controllable.

● Retain all routines and familiar pregame procedures.

● Beat Liverpool on the field.

By sharing these goals with the players, coaches can raise the players' awareness of potential distractions and insist on preparing to play in a particular way. Beating Liverpool at Anfield begins with screening out the distractions.

## Trust Yourself

Following his first U.S. Open singles championship, Andre Agassi was reported to have said he won because he finally allowed himself to play well enough to win. This confident player realized that to win big matches, he had to trust his skills. Trust, one step beyond confidence, is a vital part of those outstanding performances when players describe themselves as "being in the zone" or achieving flow. With complete trust in the ability of their bodies to meet the challenge, players can move into an automatic, virtual no-think situation that allows relaxed excellence.

Coaches can often be heard telling a player to stop thinking so much and just play. They are aware of the benefits a player can get by simply trusting the body to take over and do what is right. Trust is confidence in action.

# Coaching to Build Confidence— the Seven Key Steps

A state of confidence, a personal and collective feeling that we can get the job done, is the basis for successful performance. Many factors contribute to the process of confidence building, but key to them all is the role of the coach and the strategies he adopts. Harvard professor Rosabeth Moss Kanter underlines this: "The fundamental task of leaders is to develop confidence in advance of victory" (2004, 19).

The coach, as leader, is responsible for these elements:

- The planning, organization, and management of practice and games that act as cornerstones of confidence
- The human touches that shape a positive coaching environment that inspires and builds confidence in the players

Combined, these two responsibilities point to the seven steps a coach has to take to build confidence in his players.

## 1. Be the expert and the model.

Recently a Premier League coach resigned after a particularly disappointing performance in which his team demonstrated a lack of confidence and belief. The following factors were mentioned in the many explanations that followed:

- A feeling of not being well prepared
- Lack of conviction on team shape and tactics

- Disagreements on team selection
- Players out of position and uncomfortable
- Lack of continuity and stability
- A growing feeling that the coach himself lacked confidence and belief

However secure players are in their ability to play at that level, confidence personally and collectively will diminish if the coach does not take care of these factors. The coach's expertise—knowing what to do, organizing it, and selling it to the players—is fundamental to building the confidence of the team.

For female players, all research indicates that the coach is a significant factor in their attitudes to practice and competition—either as a positive or negative influence. The relationship between a coach and a female player is outlined by sport psychologist Gloria Balague:

> When I work with women athletes, relatedness often arises as an important motivational element. Most of the women I speak with will talk about the importance of their relationship with their coach. The personal relationship seems to be a central concern, as is having a group of teammates with whom they feel a sense of belonging. Often they feel that their coaches did not understand the relatedness need, resulting in frustration for all parties concerned. (2007, 2)

Men seem to be more able to stay motivated without positive coach support, but coaches with negative attitudes can still affect confidence. Not only must the coach be expert, but he must also model his messages on an everyday basis. Players—especially younger and female players—take their lead mentally and emotionally from the appearance, personality, and attitude of their coach. A confident coach breeds confident players.

## 2. Sell the plan.

The road to soccer success is a tough journey, and players will feel more confident if the coach presents a clear, simple, but specific map for the way ahead. Not only does this need to be presented at the start of the season but also re-presented regularly in short updates. A five-minute meeting on the field before practice can establish these factors:

- This is where we are now.
- This is where we want to go.
- This is what we have to do to get there.
- This is what we need to focus on today.

Coaches taking over teams with very low confidence can change the mood instantly if they immediately present a realistic plan to take the team forward that can be clearly understood by the players. That initial confidence boost must be followed by clear messages of the steps players need to take daily, weekly, and monthly throughout the season.

## 3. Work hard but have fun.

An element of player confidence is the feeling of being well prepared, of having done the hard work to prepare for the game. When players have this feeling, they feel they deserve to be successful; they have earned the right to win. Football coach Vince Lombardi understood this when quoting Julius Caesar:

> Without training, they lacked knowledge
> Without knowledge, they lacked confidence
> Without confidence, they lacked victory (1996, 83)

Coaches have to convince players that the hard work of preparation is not a sacrifice but an investment—both in their personal development and in the team winning games. To shape their team's confidence, the coach must prepare them for the various challenges and scenarios they might face in the game. The culture on the great teams I have worked with is one in which the players feel that no other team will work harder, prepare better, or be more ready than they are.

The best coaches, however, are clever enough to include fun as part of such preparation. The tension of being challenged every training session is fatiguing, and nothing brings back mood and energy better than some humor. Players must enjoy coming to practice—even knowing it will be hard work—and they must also leave practice with a sense of enjoyment and looking forward to the next session.

## 4. Focus on potential.

There are two kinds of coaches—those who see what their players can do and those who can only see what their players can't do. Building confidence begins with coaches seeing the potential in their players and then helping them see the same. Great coaches plant the seeds of success in their players' minds and make them feel important, appreciated, and capable of anything. Often they help players reach beyond their own self-imposed doubts, limits, and fears. Florida women's volleyball coach Mary Wise prioritizes positive and optimistic relationships:

> I work really hard at developing my players' confidence and making them feel good about themselves. When they feel pretty good about themselves, I think there is a lot they can accomplish. (2008)

## 5. Notice and reward good performance.

Confidence—a belief in players that they can succeed—is boosted when coaches notice their efforts and praise them publicly. Good coaches help players believe in themselves by stressing their strengths, always reinforcing what the player does well. Not only does this build a solid foundation of confidence, but it gives both coach and player a strong platform from which to deal with the player's weaknesses. Many coaches achieve this by using the sandwich technique:

- Praise: "Lots of good things there . . ."
- Criticism: ". . . but I think we can improve the . . ."
- Praise: ". . . and I know you have the ability to do it."

Coaches will be more likely to notice changes in performance if they have helped each player understand his role and how it fits into overall team performance. Coaches who don't work with players individually tend to notice only the mistakes. Rick Pitino, collegiate basketball coach, has a track record of building great teams by getting the best out of players:

> The most important thing I did in the course of those comebacks was to build my players' self-esteem. Don't tear them down for the mistakes that got the team in those holes to begin with; build them up to the point where they feel capable of making the plays that would result in victory. (2008, xiii)

## 6. Treat all players with respect.

Coach Alex Gibson of Manchester City Under 18 has the knack of making all his players feel like heroes. When I observe him coach, I see that he

- knows and uses every player's name;
- treats each player as a unique individual deserving special attention;
- encourages his team to express their feelings, ask questions, and come to him with problems, which he listens to carefully; and
- shows patience and understands that sometimes the best thing he can do for a young player is give him some space and time.

Naturally, Alex, qualified both as a teacher and a counselor, is highly respected by the confident young players he produces; plus his team is consistently one of the highest-ranked youth teams in the country.

## 7. Keep everything in perspective.

In my view the world is teeming with good practice coaches but lacks good game coaches. How often do we see the confidence built in training destroyed in matches because the coach lacks perspective about what he is trying to achieve? An overemotional response to a defeat can destroy confidence that is difficult to rebuild in the following week. It is very important at the end of a game to help the players know how to feel and to ensure no permanent damage is done to individual players or collective team confidence. Soccer is dominated by the psychology of results, and coaches must prepare their response to four key game results:

1. Played well and won—celebrate and enjoy.
2. Played well and lost—disappointing result, but lots of good things in the performance.

**3.** Played poorly but won—good, but we were lucky today and need to be better.

**4.** Played poorly and lost—we have to stick together, work hard, and success will come.

Coaches must be wary of their own emotional state and take great care not to say things they would later regret. Often after watching a film of the game, opinions will have changed. Don Shula, former American football coach, gives good advice: "Success is not forever, and failure isn't fatal" (1995, 4).

Coaches must also be aware of how the gender differences affect reaction to failure. A father of girls competing in swim meets put this into perspective in a personal email to me.

> What has been an eye-opener for me is to watch how each gender reacts to failure. The boys seem to take a go-it-alone attitude and go off by themselves. The girls band together to offer emotional support for a female team member to help her through the moment, hugging and even crying together. Maybe the girls' approach is more advanced. (2008)

Coaches can check their success at implementing the seven key steps by assessing themselves using table 3.4 (page 58). Clearly any criterion that cannot be assessed always needs some further thought and action. This checklist also offers coaches the opportunity to get feedback from fellow coaches, players, and parents.

## Summary

Confidence—the constant belief that challenges can be overcome—is crucial to success in soccer for both players and teams. During the course of a long, hard season, players and teams will experience varying levels of confidence as they deal with the many challenges that will occur.

Staying confident is a constant battle of positives versus negatives, and many strategies are outlined for keeping players and teams in the positive. My own role as team psychologist to Premier League and national teams can be summed up as ensuring that every day the positives drive the program, and the negatives are dealt with quickly and effectively, with everybody remaining in a state of confidence.

Players can help themselves by staying optimistic, preparing well, and remaining focused on their goals. Key to the player's strength of mind is to avoid being distracted by negative challenges, instead using positive self-talk to retain confidence and the mind-set of a winner. A strong and supportive family and friends are of great help.

The importance of the role of the coach in boosting player and team confidence is emphasized. Both in their personality and style, and the strategies they adopt, coaches have a great influence on confidence levels.

| TABLE 3.4—Coaching for Confidence: A Coach's Checklist | | | |
|---|---|---|---|
| **Coaching action** | **Always** | **Sometimes** | **Never** |
| • My leadership is based on mutual respect. | | | |
| • I am consistent in applying agreed-on rules. | | | |
| • I keep winning and losing in perspective. | | | |
| • Playing for me is fun as well as challenging. | | | |
| • All my players feel like achievers. | | | |
| • My players know I care about them as people. | | | |
| • I work hard on building positive relationships. | | | |
| • My players know I can improve their game. | | | |
| • I communicate in a positive manner. | | | |
| • My players know I will listen to them. | | | |
| • I am good at handling mistakes and setbacks. | | | |
| • I balance praise and criticism. | | | |
| • I may criticize behavior but never the person. | | | |
| • Players in trouble will come to me. | | | |
| • I see what players can do. | | | |
| • I expect my team to win. | | | |
| • I notice and reward good behavior. | | | |
| • Each player is treated as a unique individual. | | | |
| • I am enthusiastic. | | | |
| • I possess great patience. | | | |
| • My coaching creates good people as well as good players. | | | |
| • I do not let one defeat undermine our progress. | | | |
| • I am realistic but optimistic. | | | |

From B. Beswick, 2010, *Focused for Soccer, Second Edition* (Champaign, IL: Human Kinetics).

# Building Confidence at Middlesbrough Football Club

Steve McClaren and I inherited a difficult and challenging situation when we took over as manager and assistant manager at Middlesbrough. Not only did we find limited talent, but we also found that team and player attitudes had become negative and totally lacking in confidence.

With very little time to turn things around, we launched an immediate program to raise confidence levels. The following list of actions reflects that every action a coach takes has an effect on confidence, positive or negative. The list is not in priority order or in sequence—many occurred simultaneously—but each was designed with building confidence in mind:

● Steve appointed a new team of coaches (not friends) who brought expertise, experience, character, and energy. They modeled the message of winning attitudes every day.

● We recruited Gareth Southgate, a player and leader of recognized talent and character, and this sent a very positive message to the rest of the squad, the fans, and the media.

● Steve always took an optimistic approach, and he removed fear by highlighting what the team could, rather than couldn't, do and stressing the positives in every situation. He allowed every player to start the preseason as an A player and then fight to retain that grade.

● Increased communication—regular meetings, daily notice-board information, individual messages, constant interaction with the coaches—quickly led to decreased anxiety.

● We created a fresh and stimulating physical environment by such actions as reorganizing the locker room, creating a meeting and film-review room, and filling bare corridor walls with framed photographs of each first team player in splendid action.

● The coaches planned, prepared, and organized the players' daily training program with great care and attention. Doing the right thing every day was the cornerstone of our coaching philosophy, and the players responded well to the constant attention to direction, purpose, and teaching.

● Slowly we held the players more accountable for their actions and issued a player guideline handbook full of simple, clear messages spelling out how top players should live, work, and behave.

● I began a series of squad, team, group, and individual meetings designed to influence the players to think positively. This stressed that their attitude was their choice and responsibility, and while they couldn't choose every situation they faced, they could choose their response. In this way we developed a range of coping skills that helped the players deal positively with negatives.

● Wherever possible the coaches applied positive reinforcement by recognizing good performances. Even when we lost our first game at home 4-0 to Arsenal, we were able to find 15 minutes of film to show the team where we played particularly well.

*(continued)*

**Building Confidence at Middlesbrough Football Club** *(continued)*

Because our mistake-management policy was clear—no mistakes in the defending third of the field, no mistakes passing sideways or backward in the middle third, and complete freedom to play in the attacking third—we slowly removed the fear of mistakes, and our players became braver.

• Just as important as getting the right people—like Gareth Southgate—in the club was being brave enough to get the wrong people out of the club. Coaching is about bad news as well as good news, and a number of players left us in the early weeks, sending a very strong message to those who stayed behind.

• Although we built a much-improved work ethic, and practice became more intense, challenging, and meaningful, we always provided a balance of rest, recovery, and relaxation. The most common mistakes when inheriting losing teams are to overcoach and to overtrain—both of which are attitude killers.

• Finally the greatest challenge we faced in maintaining the confidence we had built was in dealing with the inevitable early defeats (we lost the first four games!). Fortunately we had prepared "what if" scenarios, and our policy was this:

  – To hold our nerve
  – To treat defeat as necessary feedback
  – To handle defeat as a one-off and not a pattern
  – To build accountability but never blame
  – To criticize behavior but never personality
  – To focus on performance and not result
  – To recognize there would be good aspects of play in a losing performance
  – To close down and move on quickly to the next challenge

The list shows that building confidence in players and teams begins with coaches demonstrating positive attitudes on a daily basis and supporting them with some well-thought-out strategies. The initiatives described here kick-started Middlesbrough to the most successful five years in their history—ever-present in the Premier League, winning the Carling Cup (the club's first-ever trophy), qualifying for European competition twice, and reaching the final of the UEFA Cup. Confidence is the foundation of all successful performance!

Not only have coaches got to organize and deliver a coaching strategy that players will commit to, but it's just as important that they not forget to build player relationships. Female players, in particular, flourish under optimistic and confident coaches who provide a positive and supportive culture.

# CHAPTER 4

# Self-Control: Discipline of Thought and Emotion

Anyone can become angry—that is easy. But to be angry with the right person, to the right degree, at the right time, for the right purpose, and in the right way—this is not easy.

**Aristotle**

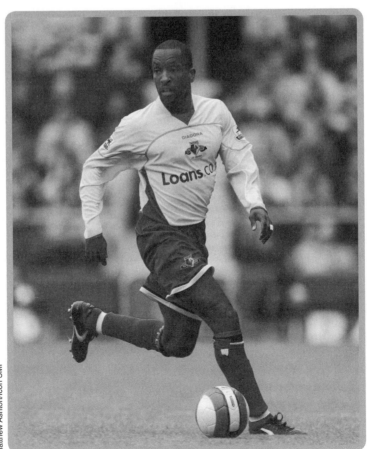

Matthew Ashton/Icon SMI

Soccer is a game of both motion and emotion. A challenging game can arouse in players a range of emotions—either empowering or disempowering. Emotional intelligence—the ability to control the self and use emotions constructively—is a vital skill of modern soccer players.

In the quarterfinals of the 1998 World Cup, England was competing well against Argentina when, in an incident of high emotion, David Beckham lost self-control and was sent from the field. Playing with just 10 men, England lost the game and their dream.

In the final of the same tournament, Brazil was expected by many to beat France. On the day of the match, however, their star player, Ronaldo, became ill, and the team prepared to play with his replacement—a well-liked senior player. Just before kickoff, Ronaldo recovered, and the decision was made to revert to the original team. Brazil took the field with a team that had changed twice on the day of the match, a coach feeling that he was not in control, and a team that was emotionally washed out. Negative thoughts, the wrong emotional state, and low energy led to a passive performance and a loss in the most important game in world soccer.

Examples like those illustrate the following:

- In a single game, players can feel happiness, sadness, fear, anger, surprise, excitement, guilt, and so on—an emotional roller-coaster ride!
- Emotions are linked with energy (*emotion* in Latin means "set in motion") and can build or drain players' energy levels.
- Self-control is one of the most important mental skills in soccer. Any loss of control will disrupt all aspects of play.

Changes in the nature of soccer have also defined the increasing importance of self-control. In the days when soccer was primarily considered a physically intimidating encounter—a war without weapons—coaches created high emotion and expected players to lose control occasionally. Changes in rules and tactics have made soccer more strategic—perhaps more like basketball. Coaches now require players who can demonstrate patience, discipline, and self-control.

The lesson to be learned from the failure of Brazil is that central to winning is the ability of each player, the team, and the coach to create a stable emotional state before the game and maintain it for 90 minutes. Players and teams who let their mental and emotional state disrupt their physical, technical, and tactical prowess will always underachieve.

Figure 4.1 shows the sequence of responses as the player reacts to soccer situations:

1. A *situation* occurs that needs to be handled.
2. The player *thinks* and defines the situation based on previous experience: "I can deal with this," or "I am not sure what to do."

3. The player *feels* the emotions associated with her definition of the situation. If the player feels comfortable, then her emotions will be positive; if uncomfortable, she will experience negative emotions.

4. The player's *energy* levels—the body's response—will be determined by emotional state. Energy-giving emotions are challenge, confidence, determination, drive, focus, excitement, joy or fun, aggressiveness, and fighting spirit. Energy-draining emotions are fear, helplessness, confusion, insecurity, weakness, depression, and self-doubt.

5. With energy available, the player will *respond* to the situation.

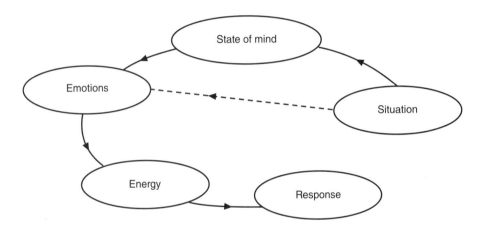

FIGURE 4.1   How players respond in soccer: the mind–body loop.

Loehr and McLaughlin (1990) emphasize the link between state of mind, emotions, and the supply of energy. They differentiate between high positive energy (energy without tension)—the ideal state for self-controlled performance, and high negative energy (energy with tension)—a dangerous state in which control is easily and quickly lost.

Figure 4.1 includes a dotted line to indicate the very dangerous moments when players react to a situation by going straight to their emotions rather than going through the proper thinking process.

This was clearly the case with David Beckham who was provoked into reacting emotionally, failed to control his anger, lost self-control, and was red-carded. I was able to work with David and the England team and could remind them that our definition of mental toughness was coming off the field with 11 players having won the game!

Much of my work with players and teams centers on shaping the attitudes and emotions that can create and maintain a state of high positive energy. By starting with a positive attitude and knowing how to apply pertinent coping strategies, the player should be able to ride the emotional roller coaster of soccer without loss of control.

## State of Mind Is Everything

How we think is how we feel, so the key to emotional control is to think positively, confidently, and calmly. The process of learning to play soccer is based on the correct mind–body coordination in all soccer situations. Coaching is preparing players, often by constant repetition, for the situations they face on the field. What coaches do not want in the game are surprises—situations not prepared for—where the players may not know what to think and fall into a negative emotional reaction.

I like Taylor and Wilson's description of this process:

> When athletes begin to experience the negative emotional chain, their thinking can become clouded with negativity that can further drive them down an unhealthy and unproductive road during competition. Athletes can alter their thinking by becoming aware of what they say to themselves and others and shifting it in a helpful direction with positive thinking (self-talk). They can also combat all aspects of the negative emotional chain by generating positive and motivating images in which they see and feel themselves overcoming the frustration, performing well, and succeeding (mental imagery). (2005, 80)

Players must work constantly to develop positive, strong, and focused thinking. Here is my advice to players:

- Take responsibility for what you think.
- Practice positive thinking.
- Never think or say "can't."
- Think more energetically—"I love soccer!"
- Stay in the present—deal with the now.
- Develop positive triggers—words, phrases, or even music—that make you think positively.
- Keep busy—avoid thinking negatively.
- Visualize only good things about your game.
- Develop positive rituals—routines that help you prepare positively for practice or games.
- Move on from mistakes quickly and get back into the positive.

Players should remember that if their feelings are negative, they only have to change the way they think: How we think is how we feel.

---

# Emotional Intelligence

Soccer will always be an emotional experience for players, either positive or negative. The problem is not with emotionality but with the appropriateness of the emotions created and their expression. Players who cannot control their emotions will find themselves fighting inner battles (for example, guilt) that sabotage their ability for focused work and clear thought. Emotion and skill execution go hand in hand. Bill Parcells sums up the problem in American football:

> A lot of kids we get nowadays have grown up macho. They can't take a dirty look, a harsh word, and they definitely can't take a slap on the back of the head from some cheap-shot artist on the other team. . . . But mature players will absorb these in their stride, even when they are out-and-out flagrant. I tell my players to put their emotions on hold—to stone face their opponent. Once the opposition knows what you are thinking, it gains an advantage. (1995, 205)

The question then is how to handle emotions with intelligence, thereby enhancing and energizing performance rather than de-energizing and disrupting it. Just as there is a sport intelligence that accelerates physical and technical learning, so too there is an emotional intelligence that embraces the skills of self-control.

Table 4.1 allows you to rate yourself and your team on how well you are managing your self-control, and table 4.2 (page 66) identifies five key stressors soccer players face and the appropriate emotionally intelligent response.

### TABLE 4.1—A Checklist for Emotional Intelligence

Assess yourself, and then your team, using these criteria:

| | Always | Sometimes | Never |
|---|---|---|---|
| Prepares emotionally for games | | | |
| Never under- or overaroused | | | |
| Able to handle the big game | | | |
| Maintains self-belief with positive talk | | | |
| Persists in the face of frustration | | | |
| Adapts easily to any situation | | | |
| Copes calmly with stress | | | |
| Can be relied on in critical moments | | | |
| Deals with other people in a mature, positive manner | | | |
| Accepts accountability for actions—never seeks excuses | | | |
| Regardless of circumstances, can be trusted | | | |

From B. Beswick, 2010, *Focused for Soccer, Second Edition* (Champaign, IL: Human Kinetics).

| TABLE 4.2—Soccer Stressors and Responses | |
|---|---|
| **Key stressor** | **Emotionally intelligent response** |
| Change | The life of a soccer player is one of almost constant change. Instead of feeling alarm, players must convert change into a new challenge and respond in a positive manner. |
| Fear | Players should understand that fear is a survival mechanism common to all people. Fear of failure helps prevent complacency. Players must learn to manage it constructively, providing the energy to meet the challenge of performance. |
| Distractions | The bigger the game, the bigger the sideshow. Players must manage this assault on their emotions and have the mental strength to get past distractions. They should strive to build a reputation of being able to play well anywhere, anytime, and under any conditions. |
| Guilt | Mistakes in soccer are usually followed by a surge of guilt and energy that players often use negatively, making one mistake into two. Players have to acknowledge that they will make mistakes in the game. They must accept each mistake as it happens, learn to let go of the guilt, and recover a positive attitude. |
| Anger | Anger is part of a player's arousal mechanism in preparing to compete. Players can use the mobilized energy positively for assertive and expressive play, or they can use it negatively and lose control. Ask players to be like good boxers—angry but never losing their temper. |

# A 12-Step Strategy for Achieving Self-Control

Like confidence, self-control is an option that players can choose. Players must decide to take responsibility for their actions and not seek excuses. Self-control strategies are based on the relationship between thought and emotion. We know that our state of mind influences our emotions, which in turn energizes our performance. So if we wish to improve our performance by controlling our emotions, we must change our thinking.

I offer a 12-step strategy to help players learn the skill and discipline of self-control, but players should only take the steps they think are right for them. Players can begin the process only when they take full responsibility for their actions.

1. Awareness. Analyze when loss of control has occurred in the past, why, when, and where on the soccer field. Identify your personal weak spots.
2. Understanding. Realize why your thinking changed and how it caused you to lose emotional balance.

**3.** Differences. Recall when you did not lose control and when you did in similar circumstances. What were the differences in your attitudes, emotions, and behavior?

**4.** Problem. Try to pinpoint the problem. For example, is it the sudden guilt of letting your team down?

**5.** Belief. Raise the expectations you have for yourself and include self-control as one of your virtues. You can change!

**6.** Reinforcement. Behavior change is accelerated by reinforcement, so you and your support group should reward improved behavior on the way to permanent change.

**7.** Goals. Set yourself a series of small goals, perhaps with the agreement of your coach, that will lead you along the route to change.

**8.** Techniques. Build a series of behavioral techniques for maintaining composure; that is, if such and such happens, then I will do this (walk away from the incident, for example).

**9.** Plan. Pursue your goals in a planned, systematic way, selecting a personal blend of techniques from those suggested in this chapter.

**10.** Progress. Improvement comes in a series of ups and downs, so be patient.

**11.** Setbacks. Accept that setbacks will happen from time to time, forgive yourself, and become even stronger.

**12.** Remembrance. Recall frequently why you are doing this and what the future will be if you don't change.

Table 4.3 indicates the self-control profile of a complete player.

## TABLE 4.3—The Complete Player and Self-Control

- Is intense without being tense
- Maintains composure and focus at all times
- Is able to handle big games as well as normal games
- Comes through in tight moments, end-of-game plays
- Makes the big play when needed
- Handles mistakes well
- Is passionate but manages anger
- Deals with other people in a mature, positive way
- Can handle the expectations of others
- Deals well with the lifestyle of a top player
- Is comfortable with success
- Can be trusted

# Techniques for Improving Self-Control

By following certain guidelines, you can improve self-control. The following techniques will be useful.

## Preparation

One of the keys to players being confident and composed mentally and emotionally before a game is the positive feeling created by good preparation. Good game preparation should result in these conditions for the player:

- The confidence he is physically ready to play
- A clear understanding of his own specific job on the field
- A clear understanding of his responsibilities on set plays, such as corners and free kicks (for and against)
- An understanding of the coach's game plan to win the game

Most situations in which a player might lose control can be anticipated by the player alone, with the coach, or with the team psychologist. By mentally playing the match beforehand, the player can tune in to the possible stressors and prepare appropriate responses to ensure control.

An experienced coach or sport psychologist can help the player understand the link between thoughts, feelings, and actions. They can review previous incidents (wherever possible I use film for this) and examine differences between successful and unsuccessful self-control. The player must look not only at behavioral performance but also at emotional performance. The player should try to recall what he was feeling during the particular incident. The player must finish such a review with a "solution bank," a set of solutions to predictable problem areas in the form of "If that happens, then I will do this."

In my first match as sport psychologist to the England under-18 team, I was taken by surprise early in the game when our star player, Michael Owen, was sent off after reacting to some close and bruising marking. I have always regretted not preparing him for a situation in which it was likely that defenders would give him special, and provocative, attention. We might have developed a mind-set for him to accept the relentless attention and use it to create space for his teammates, knowing that by showing patience and self-control early in the game, he would later have chances as defenders grew tired of chasing him.

## Relaxation

The ideal performance state for a soccer player is that of relaxed readiness, possessing energy without tension. This state allows players to stay calm, loose, and responsive to the pressures of the game. Relaxation techniques can help a player control his thinking so he can trigger emotions that remove unnecessary tension and conserve energy. Emotions are considered the windows of our physiology, and relaxation prepares the player for the critical incidents in soccer when positive thinking, body control, and energy control are part of the solution.

Relaxation techniques include stretching, breathing control, arousal management (music, video), massage, and visualization. Players who wish to develop relaxation skills should find a quiet place with a comfortable seat. They should select something to focus on, allow a passive attitude to develop, and seek to enjoy the state of nothingness. Players should try various techniques until they find one that is agreeable and then practice it so it becomes a tool they can go to instantly in moments of stress. Anxiety is often described as "information that won't go away." Relaxation, the clearing of the mind, gives the player an effective way of dealing with it and moving toward relaxed readiness.

## Performance Routines

If emotions follow our thoughts, then clearly any behavioral routines that help control our thinking will lead to better emotional self-control. Taylor and Wilson provide a useful definition: "A routine can be defined as a series of preperformance behaviors organized into a comprehensive plan aimed at maximizing the performance" (2005, 138).

When preparing to play, all soccer players are subjected to a number of factors that can interfere with their ability to perform at a consistently high level. These include their physical, mental, and emotional states; the significance of the game; and environmental and social pressures.

Attitude is a choice, and the mentally strong player will allow only positive thoughts to influence behavior. Routines support such positive thinking and minimize all negative influences. Routines put the player in control. Players should develop an active behavioral routine that keeps them busy, is familiar and comforting, and is connected to positive thoughts and emotions. Routines can be personalized from the following elements:

- Eat a favorite prematch meal.
- Check equipment.
- Arrive early, but not too early.
- Meet and greet everybody.
- Allow ample time to get organized.
- Chat with coaches and support staff.
- Avoid conversation now—focus inward.
- Listen to music.
- Get dressed.

- Keep the self-talk positive and visualize a perfect game.
- Focus on your job (see next section on trigger cards).
  - What are the three key things I do for my team?
  - How will I be a good team member?
- Ensure a good warm-up.
- Listen to the coach.
- Breathe in through the nose and out through the mouth.
- Run out onto the field and clap hands.
- You're ready to go—relax and enjoy!

## Trigger Cards

When building his self-belief, Lee Carsley (see chapter 1) was most vulnerable to doubt immediately before a game. We developed a reminder card that reaffirmed positive messages and anchored Lee's mind to a positive and assertive state:

> Be confident.
>
> Know my job.
>
> Breathe deeply—stay composed.
>
> Do simple things well.
>
> Feel good—smile.
>
> Win my battles.
>
> Relax and enjoy myself.
>
> Stay strong for 90 minutes.
>
> Seize the day—have no regrets.

At some stage before the game, Lee would find a quiet spot and read the card several times, ensuring that these were the last thoughts in his mind before playing.

## Positive Self-Talk

All players feel the anxiety of competition but differ in how they interpret what is happening to them. Whereas mentally strong players see threat as a challenge (and themselves as fighters), mentally weak players perceive it as a problem (with themselves as victims). Because players' perceptions are translated into self-talk—what they say inwardly to themselves about how they feel—they determine their emotional state. So one substitute leaves the field saying to himself, "I am a failure," and feeling anxious and depressed, whereas another substitute's reaction is "I have done my job today," and thus he feels positive and satisfied.

So one of the keys to player's mental strength in challenging situations is the ability to talk positively to himself—to be his own cheerleader. For players, positive self-talk is most under threat when playing for a coach who demands perfection and is intolerant of mistakes. Female players are keen to please their coaches, and undue pressure can quickly turn positive self-talk into negative self-talk. Coaches Shelley and Jamie Smith of South Carolina women's soccer team have a system of nonintervention during actual practice but lots of quick little get-togethers where they quietly reinforce good play. Since nobody is yelling at them, the players' self-talk—and confidence—remains positive.

Players need reminding that attitude is a choice. At the soccer clubs where I work, a player being asked, "How are you?" might respond with "I am choosing to be fine!" Positive self-talk leads to optimism, positive mind-sets, good feelings, and high energy.

## Physical Reminders

Players might use a signal—for example, a clap of the hands—to restore positive thinking when they realize they have slipped into the negative. Jacob Laursen, a former Danish international who is extremely strong mentally, ends his pregame warm-up with 10 defensive headers and then one volley clearance, which propel him into a confident and focused mental state.

## Modeling

When a player is having problems with his mental or emotional state, he can create a more positive attitude by modeling a player he admires. Mart Poom, the former Estonian national goalkeeper, models himself on the great Danish goalkeeper, Peter Schmeichel. When Poom suffers a period of doubt, he simply asks, "What would Peter do?" and gains the direction and strength to move on.

Stuart Lancaster, the head coach of the Leeds Carnegie Rugby Union team, faced a "perfect storm" of negativity in the final game of the season.

- His team had only one win all year.
- His team was already relegated.
- The opponents were the league champions.
- The newspapers had leaked the news that Stuart was leaving to take up a national appointment.

Stuart faced this dilemma before the game by presenting the players with their shirts and reminding them of the great players of the past who had worn those numbers. He asked the players to model themselves on those former heroes and produce a game worthy of them. The players responded magnificently and gave their finest performance of the season.

## Motivational Film

Generally, players love to look at sports images. Photographs, artwork, or films can capture their imagination at vital times. When the England under-18 team had to beat Russia to stay in the European championship, I asked the captain, Jonathan Woodgate, what kind of pregame meeting would most benefit our team. Jonathan recommended that we again watch the powerful motivational video *The Winner Takes It All.* We did, and we won!

The use of visual images is now commonplace at most soccer clubs. Coaches use them to arouse players, help them relax, or build their focus. For example, playing the highlights film on the team bus just before arriving at an away stadium can help distract players from a hostile environment and build positive energy.

## Visualization

Visualization is a process of internalized rehearsal during which the player re-creates her desired performance (see chapter 6). The aim is to reproduce the playing experience as vividly as possible so that a player feels she is actually playing the game. Once more the player is being put in charge of her own mind and directed to a positive focus and the banishment of negative thoughts.

Players with self-control problems should be encouraged to visualize scenes and situations that create excessive anxiety or anger. While in this state, the players must be encouraged to talk themselves out of being distracted or upset, while at the same time picturing themselves coping more productively.

## Distraction Control

If anxiety is information that won't go away, then the greatest dangers to players' self-control are internal or external distracting messages that destroy attention and trigger negative emotional response. Soccer players must learn what to pay attention to and what to ignore if they are to reach optimal focus. Examples of distracting information to be ignored are crowd noise, the opposition, negative thoughts, and thinking about past mistakes. If not ignored, these distractions can generate negative emotions and a loss of control of the performance.

Soccer is a game of read and react. Players read the ever-changing performance situation and then choose and execute the correct response. Successful players excel at both reading the game and knowing what information to ignore, which makes them unlikely to be distracted.

## Mistake Management

When I observe a soccer game, I am probably the only person in the stadium not watching the ball. I watch my team's players, especially their

# England 4, Distractions 0

At an under-18 international match in Yugoslavia, it became clear that the team could be more affected by distractions—transportation, food, hotel, training facilities, boredom, an awful pitch, and so on—than the opposition. I approached this challenge using the traffic-light metaphor suggested by Ravizza and Hanson (1995), which they developed to teach players a method of emotional self-control. This is the strategy we designed.

- Players and staff brainstormed all possible distractions so we could anticipate what was coming.
- We posted the list and checked them off when they occurred, which proved to be an amusing game rather than an irritation.
- I asked the group if distractions could beat us. "No!" they answered.
- I then asked what color would best describe our self-control if we allowed distractions to beat us. They replied that we would see red.
- If we stayed in perfect control and progressed smoothly, then we would see green.
- Once the players recognized the traffic-light metaphor, I asked how a player goes from green to red—through yellow, of course.
- We then agreed that yellow was the moment of decision, the time when we would either return to green or go on to red.
- After discussion we listed the techniques that would help us in the moments when we hovered in yellow:

  - Breathe deeply and relax.
  - Walk away to buy some time.
  - Release the tension—clap hands, stretch, and so on.
  - Recognize that a teammate needs help. The group decided that we would have a standard call, "Stay in the green." At one stage in the game, when Lee Matthews was being severely provoked, his captain, Matthew Upson, yelled to him, "Lee, stay in the green." Lee smiled, relaxed, and did not go into the red.
  - Park it until later. If a distraction occurs that we might have to deal with, but not now, we immediately park it to one side until, say, halftime.
  - Win the game. Remember that distractions help you lose.

This case study had a happy ending as England won 4-0 in appalling conditions and under a great deal of provocation. Because the players were prepared for distractions, and the team and staff had committed to staying in the green, the level of self-control was outstanding. The final message in the changing room was England 4, Distractions 0.

behavior after they have made a mistake. Nothing tests a player's self-control more than making a clear mistake—goalkeepers and strikers are especially vulnerable—in front of a large crowd.

If I have done my work properly, the player will have a recovery strategy to deal with the dangers of an emotional surge of guilt, which may cause the player to either become passive and hide, or overreact and compound the first mistake with an even worse second one. Mistakes are part of the game, so planning for mistakes is not negative thinking but positive preparation.

Middlesbrough was leading Bolton 2-0 in the 2004 Carling Cup final in front of 84,000 spectators when our goalkeeper, Mark Schwarzer, made a dreadful mistake, allowing Bolton to score. Amidst huge derision from the crowd and dismay from teammates, Mark automatically went into his mistake-management training:

- He allowed himself an emotional release—possibly swearing!
- He walked right round the back of the goal—breathing deeply.
- He kicked the far post and rubbed his gloves together, his trigger to forget the mistake and get on with the game.
- He repositioned himself for the kick off with one thought in his mind—"I'll save the next one"—and not turn one mistake into two.

In the next 10 minutes Bolton attacked relentlessly, but the refocused Mark made a number of world-class saves. Middlesbrough won 2-1, and Mark Schwarzer, after a major mistake, played a very important part in the victory.

Failure to teach mistake management leaves players without the tools they need to maintain control and prevent deterioration in performance. Players often receive yellow and red cards because they overreact to mistakes. Coaches all too often concentrate on punishing the mistakes rather than working with the player on potential corrections.

Joe Montana, former quarterback for the San Francisco 49ers, credits his former coach, Bill Walsh, with an enlightened attitude toward mistakes:

> Bill didn't jump on you for a mistake: he came right in with the correction: "Here's what was wrong; this is how to do it right." Over and over, without getting all upset, he taught the smallest details of perfecting performance. (Walsh 2009, xiv)

## Anger Management

In a highly competitive and physically challenging game like soccer, a certain amount of anger will always be present. Both coaches and players often experience anger toward the opposition, which creates an emotional surge that in people who are more accustomed to fight than flight produces a state of high energy. But anger can hinder performance as well as help it. Unless players learn to manage anger, it can produce several negative effects:

- Loss of focus: becoming blind with anger
- Loss of control to the opponent: losing focus and giving them chances
- Loss of productive play: wasting valuable time to recover
- Loss of the coach's trust
- Loss of fun and friendship: soccer becoming a battle

The following are strategies to help the player control anger:

- Identifying potential problems and the triggers that cause anger
- Preparing a response: "If this happens then I will . . . "
- Practicing nonthreatening body language
- Focusing on positive thoughts
- Stopping an undesirable chain of thoughts, recognizing and saying "stop"
- Taking calm, relaxed breaths
- Rewarding changed behavior with personal affirmations

## Role of the Coach

Coaches must understand that players need to maintain emotional control in order to perform to their physical and technical potential. Emotional readiness must be regarded as part of overall individual and team preparation to play, as illustrated by figure 4.2.

The coach must therefore plan a program that shapes and reinforces positive thinking by the players, creating an emotional state that energizes

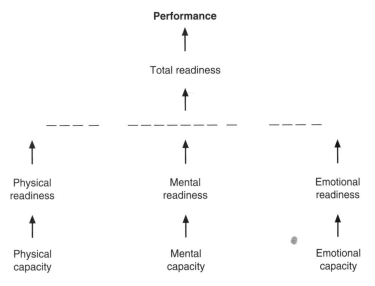

FIGURE 4.2    Balanced preparation to play.

the team to begin the game feeling a relaxed readiness. The coach cannot create a winning team unless he is willing to deal with and influence their emotional state. As one of England's former senior coaches, Colin Murphy, put it to me once, "No coach is likely to have a team of 'Steady Eddies'—it is how he deals with the 'Fiery Freds' or the 'Demon Daves' that will determine the success of his team." Coaches should emphasize the importance of emotional preparation when preparing their teams by always considering the following aspects of their coaching program:

> Are they physically ready?
>
> Are they technically ready?
>
> Are they mentally ready?
>
> Are they emotionally ready?

In considering whether players are emotionally ready, this chapter's lessons for coaches are these:

- Improve players' awareness of the importance of being emotionally ready to perform.
- Understand that by shaping the thinking of players, you will influence their emotional states.
- Be an optimistic leader; see challenges, not problems.
- When the team is performing poorly, examine the links between state of mind, emotions, and energy levels.
- Give players techniques for building self-control. If possible, use a sport psychologist.
- Be patient with younger players.
- Reinforce and reward players who demonstrate the intelligence to manage themselves emotionally.
- Find ways to understand the mood of the locker room.
- Use film, music, and other forms of communication to influence players' mental and emotional states.
- Allow the players, especially female players, to express their views.
- Prepare an emotional game plan that reviews the upcoming game and sensitizes the team to likely emotional flash points.
- Be sensitive to the nature and delivery of pregame, halftime, and postgame team talks; consider the likely emotional impact on players.
- Manage the game environment carefully to minimize distractions and avoid surprises on game day.
- Recognize and celebrate all achievements.

# Gary Learns Not to Turn One Mistake Into Two

To all outward appearances, Gary Rowett was a capable and composed defender for Derby County. In fact, Gary was sensitive and became so troubled when he made mistakes that he lost confidence and performed well below his potential. My first step was to monitor Gary's performance, with special attention to mistakes and subsequent behavior changes. Every time Gary was directly involved, I would award him a tick for a successful contribution and a cross for a mistake. After six games, we reviewed the pattern to see what it revealed about Gary's mental state during a match:

- He always started well.
- Inevitably he would make one or two mistakes.
- The mistakes would begin to affect his confidence and control.
- Mistakes would then come in clusters.
- Mistakes might even occur in the vital defensive third of the pitch.

We solved most of the problem simply by raising Gary's awareness, letting him see his performance, the pattern of mistakes, in visual form. We could link his thinking and feelings after mistakes to the resulting pattern of behavior. He immediately agreed to take responsibility for change by minimizing mistakes and, more important, by rationalizing and improving his self-control over those that would still occur. We settled on two important actions:

**1.** Gary would adopt a no-risk approach to any ball in the defensive third of the pitch, markedly reducing any chance of mistakes there.

**2.** After a mistake occurred, Gary's route back to confidence and emotional stability would be to make sure that his next touch of the ball was positive. He would select a safe option, and success with that touch would act as a release from the first mistake. He would then forget the mistake, and no longer would mistakes come in clusters.

This proved to be successful mistake management. Gary became a more mature and trustworthy defender.

Finally, coaches should reflect on their own management of emotions. After observing a youth team that was going through a difficult time, I asked permission to film a game. I concentrated the camera on the uncontrolled and negative performance of the coaches. When I replayed the film to them, they were stunned and embarrassed. Apologies followed, and everything changed from that point. The coaches learned the lesson that self-control begins with them, and they became supportive observers and analysts.

## Coach–Player Emotional Contract

Birmingham City, back in the Premier League after a long absence, faced their crosstown rivals, Aston Villa, at home for the first time in many years. With Birmingham leading 1-0 and great excitement in the crowd, a very bizarre event occurred. Aston Villa, under pressure, threw a throw-in directly back to their goalkeeper, Peter Enckelman. Not expecting this, Enckelman became confused and allowed the ball into the net.

Disaster for Villa, delight for Birmingham, and a tragedy for the goalkeeper. As the cameras focused on Enckelman's reaction to his mistake, a Birmingham fan ran on to the pitch and taunted him. The goalkeeper's self-control in such adverse conditions was outstanding, and the fan was later jailed for four months!

Birmingham won the game 2-0, and when the final whistle blew, the cameras returned to Enckelman who threw a towel over his head. Suddenly, his coach, Eric Steele, ran on to the pitch and ripped the towel off Enckelman's head, and they both walked off the field together with heads held high. The next day Enckelman, prepared by Coach Steele, faced the press in an honest and mature manner and everybody moved on. Coaches and their players are bound together emotionally, and as a result of the training and emotional support Eric Steele provided,

- Enckelman showed great self-control on the pitch.
- The Enckelman–Steele relationship and emotional contract became stronger.
- Enckelman became a stronger individual who went on to put in a string of fine performances throughout the season.

One of the questions I always ask the coach when the players leave the locker room for the field is this: "Would you change anything about the way you have prepared the team?"

Usually the answer is no, and then I say this: "Well, now you must trust them to play."

Trust is a key issue in the emotional stability of the coach–player and coach–team relationships and effectiveness. A coach must know he can trust a player, and the player must know he can trust the coach.

## Summary

Soccer is not simply a game of motion but also of emotion. Before, during, and after the game, players and coaches are challenged emotionally. Their response—with their emotions either empowering or disempowering their performance—is crucial to their success.

As players and coaches climb the success ladder of soccer, they are faced with the increased expectations of others and the dramatic consequences of failure. Emotional intelligence—the power of self-control and the ability to use emotions constructively—will become a vital skill.

Not only do coaches have to prepare their players physically and tactically for a game, but they must also prepare them emotionally. The bigger the game, the bigger the stage, and the more likely it is that the game could be defined by one moment's loss of emotional control. That is why I always remind teams before they play that real mental toughness is having 11 players, after 90 minutes, come off the field having won the game—getting sent off the field is not toughness!

Each player's emotional state, and resultant energy levels, is determined by his state of mind. Players have got to self-manage how they think and define the soccer challenges they face. Self-control must be emphasized as a characteristic of excellence.

Coaches have a vital role in helping players and teams cope with the emotional challenges of soccer. Not only must they set an example themselves of self-control under pressure, but they must teach their players the coping skills they need. Highlighted in the chapter are discussions of recovery from mistakes and setbacks, anger management, and distraction control. Emotional stability is a characteristic of consistently successful teams, and both players and coaches must focus on building the emotional intelligence and self-control to achieve it.

# CHAPTER 5

# Concentration: Direction and Intensity of Attention

When the defining moment comes along, you define the moment, or the moment defines you.

**Film,** *Tin Cup*

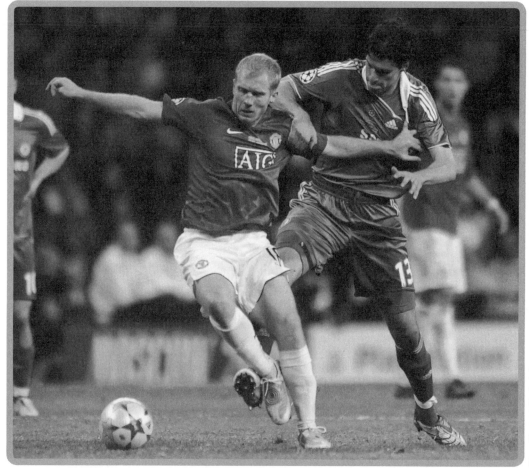

The European Club championship final of 1999 lasted for 93 minutes. As the game entered the 90th minute, Bayern Munich led 1-0, and their players had clearly begun to celebrate a great victory. One player was even waving to a friend in the crowd! Manchester United, still fully focused, seized on that lapse of concentration and scored two goals in the final three minutes to achieve a remarkable comeback. For Bayern it was truly a case of 99 percent concentration not being enough in a major final.

At the end of a 38-game Premier League season, Derby County finished in 11th place out of 20 teams. However, if all the games had ended at half time, Derby would have been champions! For the first 60 minutes of each of the 38 games, Derby conceded 24 goals—the lowest in the League. But in the final third of the game, from minute 60-90, they conceded 25 goals. Clearly Derby could defend well when fresh, but then lost focus and intensity rapidly with the onset of fatigue and anxiety.

All teams start games with good concentration levels, but each game will throw up obstacles, such as the following, to maintaining focus.

- Intrusion of negative thoughts—"what if" scenarios
- Confusion—failure to deal with changing patterns in the game
- Loss of intensity—complacent when 1-0 up and anxious when 1-0 down
- Increased fatigue—why so many goals are scored late in the game

This book emphasizes that performance follows attitude. We have already examined the importance of confidence and self-control in players' attitude. Concentration, being able to focus attention on one aspect of performance for the time necessary for success, is the third major element of attitude.

Years ago, the two strategic principles of soccer—ball movement and player movement—were limited by a combination of poor technique, a heavy ball, and slow pitches. Today's game is different; a goalkeeper's pass can initiate a goal scored in less than four seconds. Players must now deal with a transitional game of speed and variation and be able to overcome a continual unfolding of problems. Focusing skills are vital if players are to meet the challenge of a complex, fast-moving game that offers many distractions.

Ruud Gullit, the former Dutch national team player, once remarked that a 90-minute game of soccer would often be decided by one moment. Every game will contain significant situations when the player defines the moment or the moment defines the player. A lapse of focus often determines that moment. Part of shaping players' attitudes toward a mentally tough performance is helping them become aware of, and prepare for, defining moments.

## Why the Better Team Usually Wins

**Manchester United 1, Sunderland 0**

After a midweek change of manager, Sunderland had only two days to prepare to visit Old Trafford and the European champions, Manchester United.

The head coach, Ricky Sbragia, set out a 4-5-1 tactical formation in which the emphasis was on disciplined defending with quick breaks when possible.

As team psychologist for Sunderland, I gave a pregame reminder on the importance of team and individual focus for the whole of the game. The game quickly evolved into one of United dominance and Sunderland defending for their life. We came in at half-time 0-0 but warned the boys that the job was only half done. The game reached the 90th minute before United, as they do so often, created a late goal to win the game. A late lapse in focus by Sunderland determined the defining moment of the game, and 99 percent concentration caused 100 percent failure. The game statistics (courtesy of Prozone Ltd) reveal the enormous pressure United exerted on Sunderland's concentration.

|  | United | Sunderland |
|---|---|---|
| Total passes | 614 | 170 |
| Final 3rd entries | 61 | 8 |
| Penalty area entries | 25 | 1 |
| Crosses | 47 | 6 |
| Corners | 10 | 1 |
| Shots | 29 | 2 |
| Shots on target | 13 | 1 |

United's superior skill meant Sunderland defended their goal for 65 percent of the game, consistently dealing with crosses, shots, and balls into the penalty area. With so little time to rest and recover, the strain on the concentration of Sunderland, both focus and intensity, took its toll, and Manchester United seized the defining moment they had patiently worked for.

## Focusing Brings Order to Chaos

Taylor and Wilson have this to say about focus:

> [Focus is] essential to competitive success because it acts as the "director" of athletes' competitive efforts. Optimal focus enables athletes to attend to relevant cues, evaluate pertinent information, plan strategies, make sound decisions, and act in ways that will maximize competitive performance. Poor focus directs attention away from beneficial information and onto cues that distract athletes from those processes. (2005, 53)

Soccer players must learn to recognize and make sense of the flow of the game—the continuous stream of images as players and the ball constantly

## THREE KINDS OF PLAY.

1. The player who makes things happen
   - is fully focused, creative, positive, intense but not tense, and hard-working and
   - defines the game.
2. The player who sees things happen
   - is not totally involved, focuses in and out, fades out under pressure, and
   - makes concentration errors.
3. The player who asks, "What happened?"
   - lacks focus, is never in the game, is confused by too much happening around him, ball watches, and
   - sees the game pass him by.

change positions. Each player, relative to his position, must learn to focus attention on situations developing within his control while at the same time ignoring situations that are either less important or beyond control. Doing this is not easy. For some players, it proves to be the weakness that prevents progress, but anyone can develop the ability. Concentration is a habit, not a talent, and it requires motivation and constant practice.

Players will find themselves in two main situations on the field that demand different levels of focus:

1. Prime responsibility. The action of the game is in the player's area of the pitch, and he has responsibility for doing a job to help the team. The player must therefore focus totally.

2. Support responsibility. The action is away from the player, but he should be ready to provide support if needed. He can relax from total focus.

It might help players to think of their concentration like the action of a flashlight. For prime responsibility, the player must set the flashlight on a narrow beam (specific focus) with powerful intensity (high energy). This, of course, consumes considerable energy—for the light and the player—so when the action moves away, the player may switch the light to a much wider beam. The player stays informed and ready but reduces intensity to recover and conserve energy.

If a player can understand the concept of concentration—switching on to a narrow focus with high intensity and then smoothly switching off to a wider view with low intensity—then he can obtain rest when possible, begin to reduce the number of mental lapses, and start winning the defining moments.

Eric Steele, the goalkeeping coach for Manchester United, constantly emphasizes that the ability to focus is vital for a goalkeeper. Figure 5.1

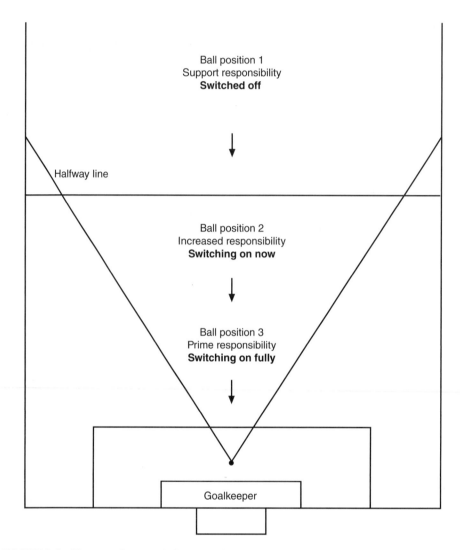

Ball position 1
Support responsibility
**Switched off**

Halfway line

Ball position 2
Increased responsibility
**Switching on now**

Ball position 3
Prime responsibility
**Switching on fully**

Goalkeeper

FIGURE 5.1  The goalkeeper's funnel of attention.

illustrates the funnel of attention, showing prime and support responsibilities, and when and where the keeper must switch on and switch off.

When the ball is in position 1, the opponent's half of the field, the goalkeeper is in support responsibility, switching off into relaxed awareness, and taking the opportunity to recover energy. As the ball moves to position 2, responsibility increases. The goalkeeper must switch on and begin to focus on the developing pattern of play. When the ball reaches position 3, shooting distance, the goalkeeper has prime responsibility, and switches on to total focus and total intensity. Nothing should distract the keeper here. So the goalkeeper demonstrates the basis of good focus—changing from narrow, focused attention when attack threatens to wide, relaxed, but aware attention when attack is not imminent.

Effective focusing is the ability to shift attention according to the needs of the particular competitive situation, so players must learn, by reviewing the pattern of the game, when they should switch on and when they can safely switch off. They must also be aware of the danger of allowing their thoughts and feelings to disrupt this process.

The development of focusing skills in players learning to play soccer is a process similar to going through the gears of a car (manual, of course!).

First gear—getting going, but shaky, too many things to think about

Second gear—making progress, but still confused, and errors are likely

Third gear—playing with more speed, but prone to distractions

Fourth gear—cruising, and becoming more focused, ignoring distractions

Fifth gear—responding automatically and in the flow physically, mentally, and emotionally

Feelings of frustration, anger, or fatigue can interfere with the process of focus. The player can find himself paying more attention to an inner world than the outer world of the game. Perhaps the most dangerous moment is after a mistake when the player inevitably has to deal with inner guilt and anger but must quickly regain focus. Teaching the player that after a mistake, the next action must be positive is another way to help regain focus and intensity.

## Good Practice Is Essential

Learning to manage focus and intensity begins in practice. Only later can players transfer it to competition. Players must accept the link between practice and competition and be willing to train at an intensity that will make transfer possible. It is foolish to train at 60 percent intensity and hope that it will transfer to 100 percent on game day. How you practice is how you play! Good coaches understand that a whole practice session cannot be conducted at full focus and intensity, but they will have two or three periods within the session when they will demand it.

Some years ago I watched an excellent coach work with young players. He organized his practice in a 60-by-40-meter space but kept one ball for each player spaced along one touch line. Occasionally he would break off from his main practice by having each boy take one ball from the touch line, dribble down the field and back, replace the ball, and rejoin him. The coach explained that this was his way of ensuring high-quality practice. When mistakes occurred, alerting him to a loss of focus and intensity, he sent the boys off on their relaxed dribble, allowing them a moment to switch off. When they returned, he could recover their intensity and the quality of practice.

Jim Taylor (1998), U.S. sport psychologist, defined four laws of training to achieve focus and intensity:

Law 1: The purpose of training is to develop effective technical, tactical, and mental skills and habits.

Law 2: Whatever players need to do in competition, they must first do in training.

Law 3: Prime training (being able to train at a consistently high level throughout a training session) requires clear purpose and prime focus and intensity.

Law 4: Consistent training leads to consistent competitive performance.

Table 5.1 identifies how to develop focus skills (the ability to pay attention to the task at hand) and intensity skills (the power and length of that attention) by emphasizing certain aspects of training.

| TABLE 5.1—Developing Focus and Intensity in Training | |
|---|---|
| **Ways to develop focus skills** | |
| Conducting realistic and demanding practice | Assessing the quality of practice |
| Preparing and teaching | Knowing what to focus on |
| Knowing when to relax the focus | Recognizing defining moments |
| Managing mistakes without loss of focus | Recovering focus after mental lapses |
| Using key words or physical action to activate focus | Using team calls that activate focus |
| Punishing loss of focus | Rewarding and reinforcing good focus |
| **Ways to develop intensity skills** | |
| Using pretraining relaxation to build energy | Building fitness levels to accommodate high intensity |
| Establishing arousal control | Using positive self-talk and being committed |
| Being prepared for and avoiding distractions | Concentrating on what can be controlled and ignoring the uncontrollable |
| Knowing when to move between active focus, semiactive focus, and relaxed focus | Recognizing when key moments require extra intensity and being able to switch on |

## Building Focus and Intensity

The ability to maintain and shift focus to meet the changing demands of a fast-moving game is a skill that can be learned and improved with practice. This section examines some of the techniques that players can use to develop that skill.

## Know Your Own Style

It is important for each player to prepare a focus routine that is both effective and comfortable. Some players favor a routine that they complete in isolation with complete control over the situation. Others prefer a routine that allows them to continue interacting with the world around them and thus be stimulated by the impact of others.

Players should select a method of focusing by personal preference and develop a routine and style they can go to when necessary. Different players can focus on or be distracted by different cues. Some are distracted by crowd noise, and some are not. Some spend the game in an internal state of anxiety, and some do not. Each player has to come to terms with her particular focusing demands and begin to develop a style of dealing with them in the game situation. The mental skills of focus and intensity are no different from physical techniques; they will become habits, and therefore automatic, only through repetition.

Such mental habits help players deal with stress situations when their focus could easily waver. The ideal performance state is often described as being automatic. Players simply release, with trust, the physical and mental habits established in practice.

## Develop a Transition Zone

Players come to practice and competition from particular home and lifestyle backgrounds. Increasingly, I have noticed that players carry focusing problems from one role to another. Basketball coach John Wooden summed up the focus and intensity that individuals need to switch on to move into the role of being a player: "When you come to practice you cease to exist as an individual—you're part of a team."

Players and clubs may find the need for a transition zone that blocks contamination and distractions from passing from one phase of life to another. This can help players focus on one thing at a time, encouraging them to switch on when they come to soccer and switch off when they return home.

Manchester United brings about this transition by starting each day with the "box"—a circle of players who keep possession of the ball from two defenders in the middle. As each player arrives on the field to start practice, they receive the yellow bib to become a defender. When this well-established routine has switched on all the players, the coach knows they are focused and ready to practice with quality.

Derby County, on the other hand, created a transitional-zone meeting room where players report to start their day. A combination of relaxation chairs, music, general and soccer-specific videos, and attitude-programming short talks all act to effect a transition in the players' minds from personal life to club and professional responsibilities, which improves their ability to focus and produce good practice. Players who wish to manage this transition individually should consider techniques such as listening to audio talks in the car, reading reminder cards with focus messages, or taking a short walk somewhere near practice where they can enter the cocoon of concentration and ready themselves to perform.

## Set Goals

Players always need to keep at the front of their minds what they want from each practice or game. Understanding their job description—what their role is for the team— allows each player to create practice and playing goals that

- focus on priorities,
- begin to eliminate distractions, and
- start to create the discipline and intensity they need to achieve.

I once coached a basketball player who, when we had a general shooting practice, would only shoot from three positions on the court. When I asked him why, he was clear that the majority of his game shots came from those three positions, and his goal was to focus his shooting skills on them.

Coaches can help by giving each practice a clear purpose and each game a specific game plan in which players have identifiable roles. If a player knows exactly what his targets are at practice and in games, it is far easier to build and develop good concentration routines.

## Conserve Energy

Maintaining focus is fatiguing, yet players must come to play with maximum energy. Returning to our flashlight metaphor, we must be sure that the battery is fully charged. Relaxation and the conservation of energy play an important part in this.

When the opportunity to switch off occurs in the game, players should take the chance to recover physically. Players should breathe deeply and let their muscles and their minds relax—I tell players to "smell the grass." Such breaks, however short, could be crucial to having the energy to focus in the vital later stages of the game.

## Always Be Prepared

A player building a focus routine needs to know as much as possible about what he will definitely have to do, or might have to do, in the game. The player can then begin creating priorities for focus and a solution bank that contains effective responses to particular circumstances.

Here are 10 questions that players must answer to be able to target full concentration:

**1.** What is my best preparation for a totally focused game?

**2.** What is my job for the team?

3. What is my job at defensive set plays?
4. What is my job at attacking set plays?
5. What must I focus on when I have the ball?
6. What must I focus on when I don't have the ball?
7. When must I be totally switched on?
8. When can I relax and reenergize?
9. What are the likely danger moments?
10. How can I help my teammates focus better?

From this information base, players may visualize the game—bringing reality forward in the mind—and build their personal focus plan. This, of course, will have to fit the team consensus on how the players prepare and build focus and intensity as a group. Table 5.2 (page 90) shows what the England under-18 team developed as their way of preparing for international matches.

## Regulate Your State of Arousal

Players must learn to check and regulate their state of arousal: too much, and they may be out of control emotionally and wasting energy; too little and they may not be able to produce the required intensity of focus and intensity. Overarousal usually occurs when the player feels threatened by the challenge he is facing. This high level of arousal hides a lack of confidence or poor focus and distraction. Coaches can help the player or team psych down by

- restating their confidence in the players,
- reframing the challenge as achievable,
- redirecting focus on to relevant cues,
- getting the players to practice controlled breathing and muscle relaxation, and
- encouraging humor to dispel anxiety.

Underarousal can result from fatigue, low motivation, or overconfidence, a dangerous situation for any player or team. Coaches should

- remind players that excellence is a habit and that good players and teams are always consistent;
- emphasize respect for opponents and remind teams that any game is losable with poor energy, focus, and intensity;
- ensure an extra-vigorous warm-up that shakes players out of their inertia; and
- if all else fails, get angry and provoke a response.

## TABLE 5.2—Preparing for Optimal Performance

**England under-18 team: Team view and response**

| The day before we should . . . | <ul><li>be positive and relaxed,</li><li>have a short practice—set plays,</li><li>be professional (i.e., lifestyle),</li><li>eat and sleep well, and</li><li>visualize our role and responsibilities.</li></ul> |
|---|---|
| On game day it's best if we . . . | <ul><li>become focused on winning;</li><li>avoid all distractions;</li><li>eat, drink, and rest correctly;</li><li>practice positive self-talk; and</li><li>turn up tune in—and be on time.</li></ul> |

**When we reach the changing room on game day**

| We must concentrate on . . . | Other players can help by . . . | We like it best when the coaches . . . |
|---|---|---|
| <ul><li>building energy and arousal,</li><li>narrowing concentration,</li><li>physical self-preparation,</li><li>mental self-preparation, and</li><li>rehearsing our jobs.</li></ul> | <ul><li>talking positively,</li><li>having a positive spirit,</li><li>respecting individuals,</li><li>communicating,</li><li>using positive reminders, and</li><li>having good humor.</li></ul> | <ul><li>talk positively,</li><li>give personal reminders,</li><li>give key team reminders,</li><li>do not talk too much, and</li><li>show no fear.</li></ul> |

| The warm-up will only work if . . . | <ul><li>everyone contributes,</li><li>everyone focuses,</li><li>there are game-related reminders,</li><li>it is enjoyable, and</li><li>it feels comfortable, not rushed.</li></ul> |
|---|---|

**In the changing room immediately before the game**

| The atmosphere must be . . . | We must concentrate on . . . | We must not think about . . . |
|---|---|---|
| <ul><li>collective,</li><li>serious but relaxed,</li><li>aggressive with control,</li><li>confident, and</li><li>professional.</li></ul> | <ul><li>building arousal,</li><li>doing our jobs,</li><li>helping the team,</li><li>getting switched on, and</li><li>feeling ready.</li></ul> | <ul><li>anything negative,</li><li>the last game,</li><li>mistakes,</li><li>injuries, and</li><li>defeat.</li></ul> |

| If we can do this our game will be . . . | <ul><li>enthusiastic</li><li>focused</li><li>committed</li><li>relaxed</li><li>energetic</li><li>collective</li><li>aggressive</li><li>bold</li></ul> |
|---|---|

# Focusing in the Game

Many things happen in a soccer game that can destroy focus and attention. This will not occur, however, if the player has mental discipline and can control her thinking in moments of crisis. Several tools can help the player develop the mental discipline to control thoughts in the game.

## Manage Anxiety

Every player will feel anxious at some stage before or during a game. Successful players are those that accept this, are aware of the signs, and have strategies to recover to confidence. Experienced players develop a performance routine (see chapter 4) that helps them stay positive during those anxious moments before the game begins. They also have a strategy for managing mistakes that deal with negative emotions by recovering breathing control, talking themselves back into the positive, and, most importantly, making the next involvement in the game a positive one.

Players will occasionally suffer mental lapses during a game, especially when fatigued, and will often use shouts or quick physical actions to shake themselves back into focus. Teammates often do this for each other with a team call that urges better concentration and effort. Sometimes players and teams can develop key words that trigger an increase in focus. These words, agreed to beforehand (see chapter 4 for the list used by Lee Carsley), can be used to raise focus levels before and during a game. Especially important is their use by team leaders at crucial moments in the game—such as defending a corner kick—when everybody needs to be at full focus. Sport psychologist Brian Miller (1997) describes how a premier rugby league team defending their try line would call the red zone to heighten concentration, emphasize low-risk tactics, and activate determined tackling.

The bigger the game, the more important good performance habits will be. If players have paid the price over the years of practice, they will have a memory bank of performance routines to deal with any situation. These should help players stay in the here and now of performance and reduce anxiety no matter where the player is performing. I once heard a ballet dancer explain how she worked hard on her steps from Monday to Friday so she could forget them when the music began for the Saturday show. Performing automatically like this produces a no-think situation—the ultimate thought control.

## Control Distractions

Loss of focus in games is often due to lack of mental discipline and focus in dealing with distractions. Distractions can create inconsistencies in performance and prevent players from achieving the level they are capable of. When players become distracted, their confidence diminishes and their performance loses momentum—they mentally go out of the game.

Many likely distractions can be anticipated and prepared for. The following strategies can help:

- Practice with intensity. When players need to be absorbed in the activity, they learn to switch off the environment.
- Practice in all weather conditions. What players are used to, they cannot cite as a distraction.
- Practice positive self-talk. Negative self-talk begins the switch off that makes players susceptible to distractions.
- Anticipate likely scenarios. Prepare by visualizing the likely distractions so players are not taken by surprise.
- Simulate distractions in practices. For example, penalty taking can be made competitive within the squad with the non-penalty takers being allowed to try to distract the player on the ball.
- Focus on the controllable elements. Players should learn to focus only on what they can control rather than diverting energy to issues they can't control—including referees!

The main thing for players to remember is that there will always be distractions, but those distractions do not have the power to influence the game unless the players let them. Mental focus and discipline are the keys to each player's performance in controlling the sideshow of soccer.

## Stay in the Now

Total focus means being locked into the here and now, but players may lapse mentally and go into the past, often because of worry and guilt about an earlier mistake, or into the future, perhaps because the mind begins to anticipate the outcome. Staying in the *now*—the present—aids the focus on incoming performance cues and also allows the player to recognize and deal with distractions.

Billie Jean King, in an article for the *London Times,* describes how she helped Martina Navratilova focus for the Wimbledon tennis final.

> All you can do is get her in the NOW. You know, when you are in that zone, the ball becomes a basketball, and time slows down. You have to be with the ball in the NOW. Don't slip into the past or the future. If she is dreaming (past or future), I bring her back into the NOW—last match I asked her to describe the wallpaper in the changing room. The trick is teaching her to do it for herself in the game. (February 7, 1994)

Players must learn to practice with intensity and understand they only have power, speed, and control in the here and now. Players, therefore, must focus on the process, not the outcome, knowing that if they take care of the present by concentrating on each situation as it unfolds, and then responding well, the outcome will take care of itself.

When Shelley Smith and her South Carolina women's soccer team were unbeaten after the first 12 games of the season and chasing the conference title (which they eventually won), I gave her the following advice based on the sport of rowing:

> Remember the rower who cannot see the finishing line and knows she can be first only if she continues to concentrate on the power, efficiency, and effectiveness of each movement that carries her away from her opponent and toward the line.

## Beat Fatigue

The great destroyer of focus in games is fatigue—physical, mental, or both—so players must work constantly on their fitness and understand how to pace a game to conserve energy when they can. When England teams played abroad in hot climates, we urged them to work smarter, not harder.

To concentrate with efficiency, players must maintain awareness and recognize game situations when they can switch between total focus, semifocus, and relaxed focus. Players and teams who do not learn this skill often pay the price toward the end of each half when fatigue hits and mental lapses occur.

## Anticipate Defining Moments

A soccer game is rhythmic in flow, each team having periods of giving and taking pressure, punctuated with sudden moments that can define the outcome of the game. Players must learn to anticipate these moments when possible and be totally focused and prepared to meet the challenge. Coaches should consider presenting to their players a short film highlighting the defining moments of the previous game. Experience suggests that such moments, either positive or negative, are often

- the opening minutes of the game, especially away from home;
- the first corner;
- free kicks in dangerous positions;
- reaction after a goal is scored;
- recovering focus after breaks in the game;
- responding to a player being sent off; or
- chasing or closing down the game in the final few minutes.

# Coaching Focus and Intensity

In my experience of working alongside coaches operating within the pressure of Premier League or national team expectations, I have seen two key destroyers of players and team concentration—overtraining and overcoaching.

**1.** Overtraining. In their desire to get maximum preparation before games, coaches often work their players too hard and too long; players then leave their game legs on the practice field. Since we know that fatigue will disrupt focus, coaches must balance work, rest, and recovery to ensure a high-energy team on game day.

**2.** Overcoaching. Again, in the desire to help the team prepare for a game, coaches fall into the trap of giving them too much information. Confusion often follows, and focus is disrupted as players try to think their way through games.

It's not what the coach knows but what the players can take, and in my experience, the best coaches aim for simplicity and clarity. Knowing where and when to pay attention, what information to select, and what information to discard in a complex and fast-moving soccer game is a mental skill that coaches must teach players. For it to become a habit that protects the player under pressure, the coach must repeat the lesson at every practice and after every game. So when developing player focus and intensity, the coach must do the following:

- Ensure physical fitness to prevent fatigue-destroying focus.
- Treat players as individuals and learn their particular style of focus and attention.
- Reinforce focus on the process, not outcome.
- Make practice and teaching relevant to game preparation.
- Give each player clear instructions on focusing priorities for his specific role, job in the team's organization, and job at set pieces (for example, corners).
- Identify lapses in game focus with each player (video feedback is useful and gives clear information).
- Give the players a game plan that reduces potential distractions and helps them structure their focusing priorities.
- Learn how to regulate arousal levels.
- Keep players focused in the present and prevent attentional drift to the past or the future.

The coach also has an opportunity to improve players' focus by managing the game environment. The coach can accomplish this on game day in these ways:

- Arranging a smooth organization to reduce potential stress on the players
- Developing routines that enhance the players' concentration
- Preventing external distractions from disrupting the process
- Creating an ambience in the dressing room (for example, with music or film) that diverts the players from internal distractions such as negative thinking and anxiety
- Not worrying if some players want to be alone
- Not interfering too much

# Summary

Soccer is a game of 90 minutes in duration, but a game can be decided in any one of those minutes. The skill of focusing is a key part of player's competitive toughness.

Concentration—being able to focus attention with intensity at any moment in the game—is learned by constant exposure in practice to challenging situations. Very often the key lessons are learned after mistakes have been made. Because so many game-defining goals are scored late in the game, it is important that coaches teach focus in practices at the point when players are fatigued.

Players need to develop a way of building their own levels of focus, switching on before practice or a game and switching off when it is over. It is important that players fully understand their roles and responsibilities on the field so it is clear to them when to fully focus on important moments. Thus players must learn how, when, and where in a game to switch on for total focus and intensity and when they are safe to switch down to relaxed but alert attention.

Coaches can help players deal with the three key killers of focus and intensity: distractions, losing emotional control, and fatigue. Dealing with these should feature in realistic practice situations. With good preparation, intensity of practice, and constant reinforcement of the importance of focus—especially in key moments—the ability to stay focused for the whole game can become a powerful strength of any team.

# CHAPTER 6

# Visualization: Picturing Success

*I never hit a shot, not even in practice, without having a very sharp, in-focus picture of it in my head.*

**Jack Nicklaus, golfer**

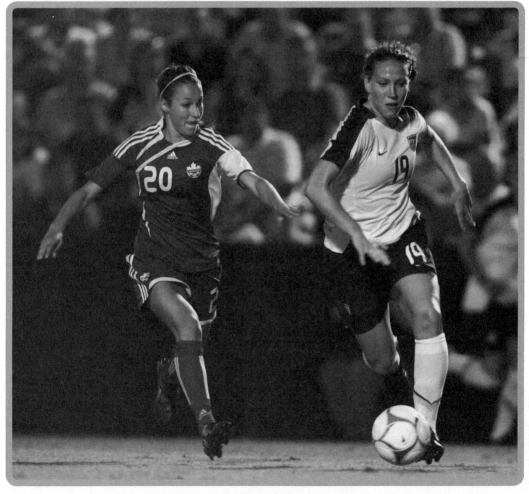

Brown University men's soccer head coach, Mike Noonan, and his team were one game away from qualifying for the 2010 NCAA championships. Due to play Dartmouth at home, Coach Noonan realized the team needed a performance boost. He asked each player to compose and e-mail to him their view of what the perfect game would be. Together, the players created an imagery script that focused on key variables such as scoring first, scoring in each half, keeping a clean sheet, no red cards, and so on. This script, cleverly reinforced by Coach Noonan, provided the stage on which the players' visualization of success became reality in a 3-0 victory!

A young and talented international player once explained to me that he had trouble sleeping the two nights before a major game because he could not stop playing the game in his mind. He was relieved when I told him I had heard the Olympic decathlon champion Dan O'Brien say the same thing. Such visualization is characteristic of many great performers. All athletes imagine themselves performing in their sport, whether running a personal record or scoring a great goal. They have found that running the possibilities of the game through the inner tape in their mind helps their preparation, especially their readiness to cope with potential stressors. They all, of course, see themselves winning and have discovered that what you see can lead to what you get. The most powerful weapon a soccer player has is the mind. Great players are those who demonstrate total control of mind as well as body.

The power of belief as a precursor to success is well documented. I advise players to read the biographies and autobiographies of the great players who have gone before them. This book constantly reinforces the importance of programming the player's software and building high levels of confidence, concentration, and composure. Coaches can do much of this for the player, but we now move to a mental skill that players can program for themselves: using visualization to develop a powerful and positive inner tape that will control physical response in times of challenge.

Biofeedback pioneers Elmer and Alyce Green beautifully described this process:

> As we begin to realize that we are not totally the victim of genetics, conditioning, and accidents, changes begin to happen in our lives, nature begins to respond to us in a new way, and the things we visualize, even though unlikely, begin to happen with increasing frequency. Our bodies tend to do what they are told to do, if we know how to tell them. (1977)

To be successful in challenging situations, soccer players need to build strong self-portraits—views of themselves as good players who can cope with whatever comes along. Visualization, using the senses to re-create or create an experience in the mind, is a process that can train the inner tape of the mind to build that self-portrait. By using vivid imagery, players can re-create the game and all its demands and develop a mental blueprint that prepares both their confidence and their strategies for coping.

# Process of Visualization

This mental skill requires the player to imagine himself playing soccer—seeing, hearing, feeling, and possibly even smelling the action. To avoid mental clutter and possible disruptions, the player should combine visualization with a state of deep relaxation. The player can then focus sharply on the imagined action. Figure 6.1 outlines the general process of visualization, and table 6.1 gives a clear example of how the player might structure the imaging process.

Jim Thompson provides an example of the former basketball star, Bill Walton, preparing himself for the upcoming game:

> He would sit in his hotel room and actually see the game and feel the movement of it. Sometimes he did it with such accuracy that a few hours later when he was on the court and the same players made the same moves, it was easy for him because he had already seen it all, had made that move or blocked that shot. He was amazed in those moments how clearly he could see the game. Moment by moment in that time he became more confident until when he arrived in the locker room he was absolutely ready. (1995, 180-181)

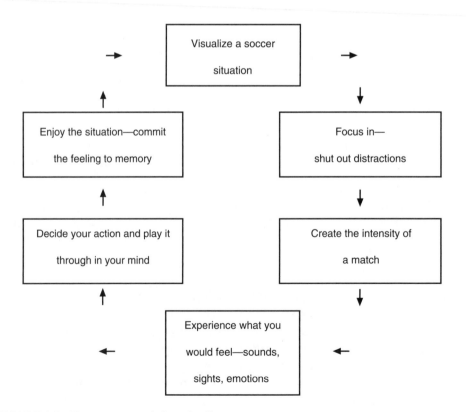

FIGURE 6.1 The process of visualization.

| **TABLE 6.1—Using Imagination to Our Advantage** |
|---|
| **Concentrate on visualizing the scene, the noise, the emotions, and so on.** |
| **1.** Get comfortable and close your eyes. |
| **2.** Feel good, confident, and proud. |
| **3.** Imagine you are in a movie theater with a big screen while sitting in a comfortable chair. |
| – You are the star. |
| – You feel good, alive, and healthy. |
| – Today is your day. |
| – You feel like a champion. |
| – You are moving well. |
| – Today is your day. |
| – Congratulate yourself. |
| – Feel proud. |
| – You know if a mistake happens, you will talk yourself back to recovery. |
| – Today is your day. |
| – You are tired but satisfied. |
| – You thank your body and mind. |
| – You know you can re-create this feeling any time you want. |

A script from Joel Fish, sport psychologist, presented at a conference of the National Soccer Coaches Association of America, Philadelphia, 1996. Used with permission from Joel Fish.

The player should strive to re-create the sight, physical sensation, sound, and smell of the soccer scene to achieve a more realistic simulation and greater benefit. The player is in effect creating an imagery script—detailed training and competitive scenarios that set the stage on which the imagery is acted out. The player will see himself in the scene, choosing the correct course of action, carrying it through with excellent effect, and even hearing the approval of the crowd and positive comment from the coach. The key to visualization is that a positive image of this particular situation now exists in the player's memory. The player can then access it when a similar situation occurs in a match. At the very least, by having something to draw on, the player will not be caught completely off guard.

Visualization is a process that players can apply at any time, but here are the key moments:

● Before, during, and after practice, to rehearse the upcoming performance
● Before competition, to relax and review the game plan

- During competition, to rehearse movements and events before they occur
- After competition, to evaluate good and bad aspects of performance

The more a player practices visualization, the more accurate the images will become. The memory trace will become stronger, the image more accessible, and the emotional support more powerful, boosting both motivation and confidence.

## Benefits of Visualization

Players and coaches who use visualization believe it helps them to

- improve skill learning and performance,
- perceive strategy better,
- reinforce self-belief and see themselves as winners,
- learn self-control and develop coping strategies,
- practice mentally what they experience in the game,
- learn to focus and shut out distractions,
- improve relaxation,
- link mind and body to produce the appropriate energy state, and
- recover from injuries.

To maximize benefits, players should employ the following approach:

- Relax; a calm state of mind is essential.
- Use all the senses; the stronger the imagery, the greater the chance of success.
- Visualize in the positive, always seeing or feeling you are playing well.
- Focus on the process; do not go directly to the desired outcome (a snapshot) but imagine the whole process leading up to the performance (a movie).
- Be specific; see all the details clearly, leaving nothing out.
- Show belief by being committed to visualization and believing that what you see is what you get.
- Be patient; it will be a while before you see benefits, but short, consistent sessions will lead you there.

## Using Visualization to Improve Performance

Although visualization can be used for any performance issue the player or coach would like to rescript, the process has been applied to good effect in specific instances.

## Skill Learning and Practice

It has often been demonstrated that the best kind of learning is a combination of visualization (mentally rehearsing the movement and thus programming the software) and physical practice (programming the hardware). Professor David Gilbourne of Liverpool John Moores University advocates that players develop imagery scripts in which they visualize in detail the stimulus–response procedure of a particular skill on the pitch (see table 6.2). In this written account of the visualization practice, the player would be required to pay great attention to all the details involved in the image:

> For example, a typical script may include references to situational factors such as other players, the ball, the feel of studs in the ground, the noise of the crowd, the sense of movement, changes in the muscular tension as a player recalls accelerating, twisting, jumping, or landing, an awareness of accompanying emotions, and so on. (1999)

| TABLE 6.2—An Imagery Script for Technical Development |
| --- |
| Technique: Crossing the ball at pace and hitting to the far post. |
| **Stimulus propositions** |
| **1.** I see the defender trying to force me infield. |
| **2.** I hear the center forward shouting, "Take him on." |
| **3.** I see the ball at my feet and my knee over the ball. |
| **Response propositions** |
| **4.** I feel my shoulder dip as I fake an inside move. At the same time my left foot pushes the ball forward. |
| **5.** I drive hard with my right leg, feel the ground under my boot, and feel my arms drive (as I accelerate after the ball). |
| **6.** I think, "Cross with pace." |
| **Stimulus propositions** |
| **7.** I glance into the penalty area and see Steve peeling away from the far post. |
| **8.** I switch focus onto the ball. |
| **Response propositions** |
| **9.** I think, "I have to lift the ball over the defender." |
| **10.** I adjust my stride and feel my legs hit the right tempo and rhythm. |
| **11.** I feel my body lean away and whip my left foot around the ball. |
| **12.** I feel my body overbalance as I watch the ball arc into the penalty box. |

Reprinted, by permission, from David Gilbourne, 1999 (Spring), "Using imagery to enhance technical development," *Insight: The Football Coaches Association Journal*, volume 2, issue 3.

## Understanding Tactics and Strategy

To perform well, a player must understand the tactical shape of the team and her role within it. When a team must change tactics quickly and significantly—as often happens with national teams playing tournament soccer—the only preparation available may be to take the whole team through a visualization process that uses the form, "If this happens . . . then we will . . ."

One of the teaching methods I have used is to gather the team around a tactics board and then ask questions. With both teams lined up on the board in their correct tactical shape, I would ask the captain to "kick off" for our team, decide where the ball will go, and then move the pieces on the board to reflect that. The next player might be told that a free kick has been awarded against us and asked to show our defensive positions. Other questions could deal with a counterattack, a corner, a direct free kick, having a player sent off, and so on. Players can also be asked to visualize how the team should react when the opposition suddenly changes tactics.

## Warming Up Mentally

Players have many ways of warming up mentally for a game. Most include some form of visualization—rehearsing the game in their minds. Players often sit quietly and mentally rehearse the focus they need for their first involvement in the game: first touch, first tackle, first header, and so on. I often tell strikers that their first touch may be the best opportunity to score in the whole 90 minutes—so be ready! Players can also try to capture on a reminder card the essence of their game in 8 or 10 words or short phrases and then read it just before the game.

## Rehearsing Performance Routines

Although players often play on automatic, letting their habits take over, in situations such as penalties, corners, and free kicks, players have time to think and can therefore rehearse their actions. An increasingly important aspect of soccer is the penalty shootout. Although it is impossible to reproduce the shoot-out exactly on the practice field, with visualization we can prepare the players' minds for the surge of emotion and help them create disciplined performance routines that they can hold on to. Then on that long walk from the center circle, they can be rehearsing an approved routine that not only helps them avoid distractions but also boosts confidence at a vital time.

## Managing Stress

All players feel stress, but successful players learn to cope with it. Some even learn to thrive on it. With players who are susceptible to stress, I use visualization as a way of rescripting emotional expectations. When such a player visualizes a challenging game, she normally sees moments of potential stress and negatively programs the inner tape. A coach, sport psychologist, or fellow player can change this picture by reminding the player of her ability, experience, past success, strength of the team, and so on.

I often ask a player, "What's the worst thing that can happen—and can you live with it?" The best visualization involves feelings, using the following imagery pattern:

- What if this (potential source of stress) happens?
- How will I feel?
- Then I will . . .
- And therefore I will regain control.

So, for example, a player receives a yellow card, feels angry and guilty, but remembers to stay out of further trouble for the sake of the team, and therefore regains control. Relaxation techniques such as meditation and yoga can aid this entire process.

## Building Confidence

Clearly, the more a player sees himself as a winner, the more likely he is to perform that way. Coaches must find ways to remind players how good they can be (not how poor) if they want them to have the inner strength to face competitive challenge. The message must be strong enough that eventually the image becomes reality. At Middlesbrough, I helped turn around a somewhat critical culture to one based more on positive reinforcement.

### Pele Prepares Mind and Body

The great Brazilian player Pele had a pregame routine that never varied. One hour before the game Pele would find a quiet place to relax. Stretched out and comfortable, he would begin visualizing his background of playing soccer as a youngster on the beaches of Brazil. He would use all his senses to recapture the moments when he had so much fun. Pele would then switch his thinking to recall the greatest moments in the World Cup, reminding himself he was a winner on the big stage.

Then he would switch to the game coming up and see himself performing at the highest level: beating defenders, making great passes, and scoring goals. After half an hour spent filling his mind with this slide show of positive images, Pele turned to his body and stretching exercises. By the time he entered the stadium, Pele knew he was physically and mentally prepared.

Players were encouraged to see and feel themselves performing well before the actual game and to increase positive self-talk. We supported this with highlight film clips that featured all the players doing things well. Players with strong self-esteem are far more likely to receive criticism of performance without damage. Their inner tape will still show them as winners.

## Recovering From Injury

A sudden injury—and the resultant withdrawal from the excitement and involvement of team participation—can often damage a player psychologically as much as it does physically. As always, the player has a choice about how to regard the injury.

- The player may take a negative view by thinking, *This is awful.*

- The player might be more positive and say, "Unfortunately, this has happened. How soon will I be back playing, and what do I have to do?"

Positive imagery has been demonstrated (Taylor and Wilson 2005) to aid the healing process by reducing muscle tension, increasing blood flow, and stimulating strength gain. The player's support group—coaches, medical team, other players, and family—has the job of encouraging the player to visualize the injury and rehabilitation in strong, positive ways. Although the player cannot practice physically during rehabilitation, visualization promotes some maintenance of skills during recovery.

## Managing Energy

The mind and the body are so strongly linked that when a player visualizes an action, the body begins to prepare a response. If the player learns to visualize positively, the body will prepare for action in a positive manner with increased energy. Players who visualize negatively will experience the reverse. So how players think influences how they feel, which in turn generates their potential energy state. Coaches who are aware of this effect will be careful to present players with messages and images about the next game that evoke the required visualization and therefore induce the correct energy state. Figure 6.2 shows that the most successful players, those who visualize positively, will be in a state of high positive energy.

This describes exactly the feeling of relaxed readiness, a state of high positive energy, that we try to produce in our players just before game time. Players who are complacent or not fully aroused will find themselves in a state of low positive energy, a relaxing place but not what is needed for winning. Without proper mental preparation, a team, having taken the lead, may be thinking to themselves, *The pressure is off, so relax.*

| | Player images → | Emotional state → | Energy state → | Performance state |
|---|---|---|---|---|
| **A** | –The winner<br><br>–The best<br><br>– In control | – Excitement<br><br>– Happiness | – High<br><br>– Positive | – Activated<br><br>– Committed<br><br>– Confident |
| **B** | – Unhurried<br><br>– Easygoing<br><br>– Relaxed | – Contented<br><br>– Calm | – Low<br><br>– Positive | – Passive<br><br>– Unmotivated<br><br>– Vulnerable |
| **C** | – Irate<br><br>– Frustrated<br><br>– Revengeful | – Anger<br><br>– Excitement | – High<br><br>– Negative | – Destructive<br><br>– Damaging<br><br>– Out of control |
| **D** | – Depressed<br><br>– Powerless<br><br>– Tired | – Fear<br><br>– Sadness | – Low<br><br>– Negative | – Passive<br><br>– Unwilling<br><br>– Victim |

**FIGURE 6.2** The effect of visualization on a player's energy and performance.

Players who don't care or feel overwhelmed will produce low negative energy. Coaches hired to turn teams around often find their new teams in this state. Changing the way the players visualize themselves and their situation is an immediate priority.

Finally, the most dangerous energy state is high negative, where players find themselves in uncontrolled passion, negatively burning up energy. When a team or player is not mentally disciplined, an adverse incident in a game or even pregame can throw them completely out of control—misuse a burst of high energy—and reduce the chances of winning. Coaches often use anger to inject energy into a team, but they must ensure that the player or team is mature enough mentally to channel it in a positive direction.

# 10 Ways Soccer Players Can Use Visualization

Following are 10 ways that players can rehearse mentally to improve their performance.

1. Seeing themselves playing well—in their minds or on film—motivates players.

2. Seeing potential success persuades players that the repetitive nature of practice is worthwhile.

3. Thinking through a practice helps the player to better acquire skills.

4. Imagining how admired players would react often influences players' behaviors.

5. Thinking through and rehearsing tactical situations—for example, an attacking corner—can help players clarify their roles and responsibilities.

6. Reviewing the upcoming game and imagining a successful performance can help build confidence and generate positive emotions—and therefore, energy.

7. Imagery of upcoming competitive situations can also help players prime their focus and intensity to competitive levels.

8. If players during the course of the game begin to feel negative, a short burst of positive imagery during a break in the game can restore a positive and winning attitude.

9. Although players on the bench are not physically involved, they can maintain involvement and focus by studying the game and mentally rehearsing their options.

10. After the game, and when alone, players can replay important parts of their performance to identify strengths and weaknesses and determine what changes needed to be made.

## The Chris Powell Story

Chris, a talented and mature fullback at Derby County, was asked to extend his normal defensive role to that of a wingback, therefore having an attacking assignment as well as defending responsibilities. Chris was clearly failing to make this change when he came to see me. Through discussion, consultation with the coaches, and video analysis of Chris in action, it became clear that he was physically and technically capable of being an outstanding wingback. Equally clear was that he couldn't commit mentally or emotionally to the position.

I encouraged Chris to use the process of visualization to imagine scenes from games in which he would be playing as a wingback. From this we began to identify an accurate job description that encompassed all the physical, technical, and tactical demands, and the thoughts and feelings Chris associated with each of these demands. We were able to establish that the problem was one of confidence and assertiveness. For Chris, defending was a science that allowed him to exert maximum control, whereas attacking was a gamble with increasing risk. Therefore, his confidence and assertiveness drained away as he crossed the halfway line to join the attack.

So we began a process of helping Chris mentally simulate—by private visualization, discussion, and video review—the movements, thoughts, and feelings linked with positive attacking from a wingback. We always emphasized that Chris should develop an image of a successful attacking play and try to involve all the senses that accompanied the action. We monitored progress through weekly analysis and observation of the contributions Chris made in the attacking half of the field. The coaching staff and I offered praise and reinforcement for progress.

Slowly we removed the mental and emotional barriers in his mind and reinforced his belief that he could make the change. Chris began to show much greater confidence and assertiveness when attacking. Instead of hiding, he began to demand the ball. Chris overcame the problem, scoring two goals in the Premier League, and being elected club Player of the Year, demonstrating that players can mentally shift gears to undertake new responsibilities on the pitch. Visualization is one of the tools at a player's disposal. Clear the mind, and the feet will follow.

## Summary

Visualization is a mental tool that some players and teams find helpful in preparing their minds to meet the challenge of the game. A clear link has been established between positive thinking and the likelihood of positive action, so players are encouraged to spend time visualizing themselves performing with excellence. What you see is often what you get.

Such mental imagery allows players and coaches to spend thoughtful time consistently working on areas they need to improve. Players can systematically visualize their development of the technical, tactical, and mental aspects of their game. Such a program is best when organized and scheduled for the same time every day as part of the daily training routine.

Visualization is recommended for building confidence, developing strategies to cope with stress, understanding tactics and strategy, and assisting the recovery from injury. Of great importance is the link between visualization—how we see ourselves—and our emotional state, our energy state, and, therefore, our potential for performance. As we exercise the mind, it grows stronger. The more the player pictures success, the more energy is created to achieve it.

# CHAPTER 7

# Mental Toughness: Disciplined Thinking, Disciplined Action

Being better than your opponent at coping with the many demands and staying more consistent in remaining determined, focused, confident, and in control under pressure

**D.F. Gucciardi, sport psychologist**

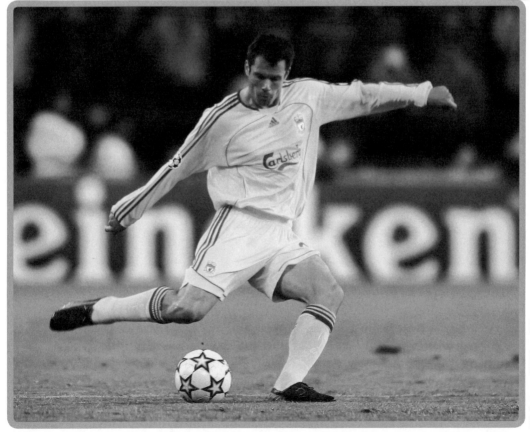

The best example of mental toughness I have seen on the soccer field came during a Champions League semifinal. Manchester United, needing to win, had travelled to Italy to face a Juventus team who had not lost a European championship match at home for 14 years. Despite the intimidating atmosphere, and despite conceding two goals in the first 12 minutes, United stayed tough, stayed in the game, and won 3-2.

Although I was impressed by the mental toughness of the United team, I was more impressed by the character shown by Roy Keane and Paul Scholes. Both had to play the game knowing that if they received a yellow card, they would automatically miss the opportunity to appear in their first European Cup final. Neither player accepted this as an excuse to limit their performance; instead, they committed physically and mentally to a great team victory. The real mental toughness, though, emerged after both received yellow cards. Neither player used missing the final as an excuse to lower the intensity of their playing. In fact, they actually stepped up their game and demonstrated disciplined thinking and action for the whole ninety minutes – real mental toughness in action!

Of course, all human activities are challenging, but being successful at soccer, an activity that publicly labels players as winners or losers, requires great mental and emotional strength alongside physical and technical excellence. A youth soccer team that easily wins all its games will be highly praised, but the players will be mentally and emotionally unprepared when they move up a level and start to lose games. The mentally tough player must be able to live with insecurity, treat setbacks as part of the price to be paid, and withstand what may seem like constant criticism. In Barrell and Ryback, Mark Price, former NBA basketball player, describes how his tough mind-set dealt with failure.

> I am not afraid of pressure. People remember the five or ten shots that Michael Jordan made at the end of a game to win, and they don't remember the fifty he missed. If you calculate it, the chance of hitting a shot at the end of a game is not very high. Some guys are afraid to take that chance. They don't want to be a hero unless there is a 100% chance, and they don't want to take any chance of being the goat. I am willing to be the so-called goat for a chance to be a hero. Getting the ball in "crunch time" is exciting and challenging. I am thinking, "Hey, I can make it and I am going to take it. If I don't make it, well at least I gave myself a chance" (2008, 121).

Coaches often complain that young soccer players lack such toughness. A changing and less challenging upbringing can leave young players unprepared to meet the challenge of competitive soccer. In her book *Nation of Wimps: The High Cost of Invasive Parenting* (2008), psychologist Hara Estroff Marano describes the dangerous outcome for young people of modern overprotective upbringing. I summarize her conclusions in the following list.

- No sense of self
- Lack of independence
- Fear of risk or failure
- Inability to handle difficult situations
- Reluctance to lead, take responsibility

So coaches are faced with developing an environment for practice and competition that teaches players to first cope and then thrive on the pressures. Such toughness training is explained by sport psychologists Loehr and McLaughlin:

> Toughness training is the art and science of increasing the talented player's ability to handle all kinds of stress,
>
> - physical,
> - mental, and
> - emotional,
>
> so they become an effective competitor. (1990, xvii)

Coaches are still seeking players with talent and attitude, but they recognize that the limiting factor for most players as they advance will not be talent, but mental toughness. There are many, many players playing at the highest levels of soccer who would not score an A on talent, but their A attitude drives them to success. *USA Today* (February 2004) set out to select the 10 toughest athletes in U.S. sport. Their conclusion was that toughness was both physical and mental.

*Physical toughness includes these elements:*
- Courage, confronting opponents aggressively
- Dealing with physical punishment, abuse, pain
- Handling injuries, recovering quickly
- Preparing hard, training beyond the norm
- Durability, playing every minute, every game

*Mental toughness includes these elements:*
- Being brave, always wanting responsibility
- Having a competitive attitude in games and at practice
- Staying optimistic and positive in all things
- Being confident, with a high sense of self-belief
- Having resilience, always bouncing back
- Taking risks, if it means having a chance to win
- Being demanding, seeking high standards from teammates
- Staying focused, ignoring distractions
- Being single-minded, never quitting
- Staying a learner and taking failure as feedback

Table 7.1 (page 112) allows coaches to make a general assessment of the mental toughness of their own players. Please read this chapter before completing the assessment and remember to score within the context of age, gender, and level of competition.

Coaches should not rely on just their own assessment but try to check this against the views of the player and other coaches and support staff working with the team.

Any player scoring over 84 shows very satisfactory mental toughness, and coaches need only to encourage and maintain this. For those players 60 to 83 (average), more analysis is needed, and coaches should examine particular areas of weakness and devise an action plan to remedy them. Below 60 reflects players with a weak attitude, and coaches must review the player's ability to deal with the challenge of soccer.

## Mental Toughness Is a Winning Attitude

Throughout this book are numerous examples reinforcing the principle that performance follows attitude. Thus the starting point for a player or team wishing to become mentally tougher has to be creating a positive and winning attitude. Mental toughness is the ability to perform physically what a player is committed to mentally. If that commitment wavers because of a setback, then clearly performance will be a step closer to failure.

Failure to establish mental toughness is almost always a problem of the player getting in her own way mentally. Each player has a personal battle to fight deciding whether her internal dialogue will be positive, "I can," or negative, "I can't." This is especially true for those players who have

### Mental Toughness Is Coming to Compete Every Day

While recovering from an injury, Paul Scholes, a Manchester United star, needed some active involvement, but only the under-17 squad was training. The club physiotherapist, Rob Swire, asked the under-17 coach, Neil Bailey, "Can Paul join in?"

Neil readily agreed, and when he later came back into the coach's room, he reported that Paul had put on a "master class" in every phase of the practice. Paul never gave the ball away, received it twice as much as anybody else, provided a number of assists for goals, scored goals, and won every race in both the warm-up and team run at the end of training.

For Paul this was the most natural thing in the world: he comes every day to compete, to excel, and to prove himself yet again. For him excellence is a habit; he can't switch it on or off. He's a true example of mental toughness. For coach Neil Bailey it was a brilliant opportunity to gather his lads in—after they clapped Paul off the field—and point out that everyone now knew the standard it takes to get into the Manchester United first team!

## TABLE 7.1—Assessing a Player's Mental Toughness

**Player's name**

**Motivation: level of intrinsic motivation and determination to succeed**

| Not motivated | 1 | 2 | 3 | 4 | 5 | 6 | 7 | 8 | 9 | 10 | Very motivated |
|---|---|---|---|---|---|---|---|---|---|---|---|

**Confidence: level of self-belief**

| Self-doubt | 1 | 2 | 3 | 4 | 5 | 6 | 7 | 8 | 9 | 10 | Self-belief |
|---|---|---|---|---|---|---|---|---|---|---|---|

**Optimism: level of optimism about all things**

| Very negative | 1 | 2 | 3 | 4 | 5 | 6 | 7 | 8 | 9 | 10 | Very positive |
|---|---|---|---|---|---|---|---|---|---|---|---|

**Focus—capability to stay focused and avoid distractions**

| Easily distracted | 1 | 2 | 3 | 4 | 5 | 6 | 7 | 8 | 9 | 10 | Very focused |
|---|---|---|---|---|---|---|---|---|---|---|---|

**Competitiveness—extent of competition at all times in all things**

| Easily beaten | 1 | 2 | 3 | 4 | 5 | 6 | 7 | 8 | 9 | 10 | Very competitive |
|---|---|---|---|---|---|---|---|---|---|---|---|

**Consistency—level of performance maintained**

| Very inconsistent | 1 | 2 | 3 | 4 | 5 | 6 | 7 | 8 | 9 | 10 | Very consistent |
|---|---|---|---|---|---|---|---|---|---|---|---|

**Emotional control—level of discipline under pressure**

| Uncontrolled | 1 | 2 | 3 | 4 | 5 | 6 | 7 | 8 | 9 | 10 | Very controlled |
|---|---|---|---|---|---|---|---|---|---|---|---|

**Resilience—ability to bounce back from setbacks**

| Fragile mind-set | 1 | 2 | 3 | 4 | 5 | 6 | 7 | 8 | 9 | 10 | Very resilient |
|---|---|---|---|---|---|---|---|---|---|---|---|

**Learner—response to failure as a lesson for improvement**

| Nonlearner | 1 | 2 | 3 | 4 | 5 | 6 | 7 | 8 | 9 | 10 | High learner |
|---|---|---|---|---|---|---|---|---|---|---|---|

**Challenging—expected performance quality from teammates**

| Nonchallenging | 1 | 2 | 3 | 4 | 5 | 6 | 7 | 8 | 9 | 10 | Very challenging |
|---|---|---|---|---|---|---|---|---|---|---|---|

**Pressure—level of performance when it really counts**

| Chokes | 1 | 2 | 3 | 4 | 5 | 6 | 7 | 8 | 9 | 10 | Responds well |
|---|---|---|---|---|---|---|---|---|---|---|---|

**Ally—either their own best ally or worst enemy in games**

| Enemy | 1 | 2 | 3 | 4 | 5 | 6 | 7 | 8 | 9 | 10 | Ally |
|---|---|---|---|---|---|---|---|---|---|---|---|

Maximum total score: 120
Player's score:

| Mental toughness rating: | 96-120 | Very high |
|---|---|---|
| | 84-95 | High |
| | 60-83 | Average |
| | 36-59 | Below average |
| | ≤35 | Help! |

From B. Beswick, 2010, *Focused for Soccer, Second Edition* (Champaign, IL: Human Kinetics).

a tendency to lose self-belief and confidence over mistakes and setbacks. For them, maintaining mental toughness can be an everyday problem. Players must remember the advice of the great boxer Muhammad Ali: "Never come second best to yourself."

Players and coaches must create a training and competition culture that constantly shapes the state of mind in a positive and confident way. Mental toughness is a state of mind that players can develop by applying the following principles:

- Think like a winner. Show high self-belief and expect to win.
- Turn negatives into positives. Treat setbacks as an inevitable part of the challenge, and learn from them to become a more complete player.
- Deal with the unexpected. Regard demanding, changing conditions as the ultimate challenge; enjoy being tested and believe that "tough times don't last, tough people do."

We have already established that a positive state of mind leads to positive emotions and the high energy needed for successful performance. Table 7.2 illustrates the same process, albeit a little simplistically, with an example of how two players—one mentally tough, the other not—might react to a missed chance of scoring.

### TABLE 7.2—Mentally Tough Versus Mentally Weak

Comparison of a mentally tough player with a mentally weak player after missing a good chance to score

|  | Mentally tough | Mentally weak |
|---|---|---|
| **Attitude change** | Thinks, "I'll get the next one," remains positive, and does not lose self-belief | Thinks, "I'll never score now," becomes instantly negative, and loses all self-belief |
| **Emotional response** | Remains enthusiastic, stimulated, and vigorous | Becomes irritated and discouraged, loses hope, and blames others |
| **Resultant energy state** | Remains positive in direction and high in intensity | Becomes negative in direction and low in intensity |
| **Effect on performance** | More likely to recover well and score with a later chance | Becomes increasingly passive, hides, and is more concerned with not missing again than working for another chance to score |

# Four Steps to Mental Toughness

The ideal performance state and the mental toughness we seek are characterised by a clear sense of purpose and direction, a degree of resilience, emotional calmness, and the fuel of high positive energy. The following steps, then, should become essential elements of players' training and competition routines.

## Step 1: Develop a Strong Self-Identity

Our performance is often the result of our expectations, so unless we think and feel like winners, we are unlikely to perform like winners. Players should check themselves for the following practices, which can help develop a winning state of mind:

- Remember you are already a winner—recall all your previous successes.
- Always look good—reflect the image of a winner.
- Control your thoughts and allow only positive self-talk.
- Be your own cheerleader—reward yourself at every sign of progress.
- Become more assertive in imposing yourself on the situation.
- Take responsibility for your actions—excuses are the first signs of weakness.
- Be persistent—do not accept failure too easily.
- Make confidence a habit—don't fluctuate between confidence and fear.
- Keep learning—the battle is never won.
- Copy role models to help develop positive, winning behaviors.

When coach Tony Pickard helped convert tennis star Stefan Edberg from an anxious loser to an assertive winner, he used a combination of positive self-talk and confident body language: "Fix the body language and the mind stands tall."

## Step 2: Become and Stay Motivated

The most important question a player must answer is why he commits to the challenge, accepts the criticism, and deals with possible failure. It takes courage to cross the white line at the start of a match. A player can reach that level of arousal only by being fully motivated. Commitment to play is a choice, and nothing can affect performance as dramatically as a sudden loss of motivation. Without motivation and without the drive to achieve, the player cannot develop the mental toughness to survive the challenge of soccer. Problems become barriers, not challenges.

After working with the England national women's team, I became more aware of how difficult the choice of playing soccer can be for women players. Figure 7.1 shows that throughout a woman's soccer career, in the important period from 11 to 34 years of age, she will continually face the dilemma of choosing between the potential rewards of soccer and social and family life. My advice to the coaches was to introduce more in-depth communication, reminding the players constantly *why* they make the commitments (the rewards) before detailing *how* they must pay (the costs). In an interview for *Championship Performance,* women's ice hockey coach Mark Johnson supports this strategy:

> With women, their communication skills are a little more in-depth. For example, they may want a greater explanation of why we are doing something. Instead of just diagramming it or demonstrating it, they want you to explain why you are going to do it. That ties in with the motivational, because now they understand why they are doing a particular drill, and they see how it fits in to the bigger picture of our success. (2007, 1)

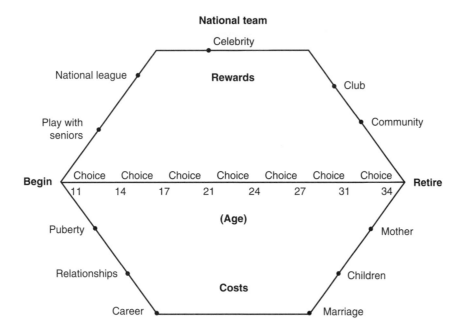

• Critical points

FIGURE 7.1 Rewards versus costs at various stages of a female player's career.

The sources of motivation are both intrinsic and extrinsic. A mentally tough competitor will be self-motivated and self-directed. This player is involved because she wants to be. Figure 7.2 identifies how the player's motivation must move through certain stages or challenges before becoming an intrinsic element of mental toughness. In the early stages, family and friends motivate players. Players then move on to the more critical influence of the coach. Of course, many players do not survive these stages and drop out because they lack either physical ability or mental strength.

The final stage, when motivation switches from extrinsic to intrinsic, is the point at which mental toughness becomes critical. The player is now driven by comparisons with players she admires and a desire to perform to potential. Rather than relying on the views of others, the player now checks her performance against personal standards. Although not isolated from external influences, the player now controls her state of mind and is much tougher mentally.

It helps, of course, if the player's social support group is positive and supportive in the journey to excellence. Although male players benefit from both intrinsic and extrinsic sources of motivation, women soccer players may not receive complete social support at certain stages in their development. The "spinning plates" example I include on the next page made me very aware of the many roles and responsibilities they face and the strain that time and effort on soccer may bring to both family and friends.

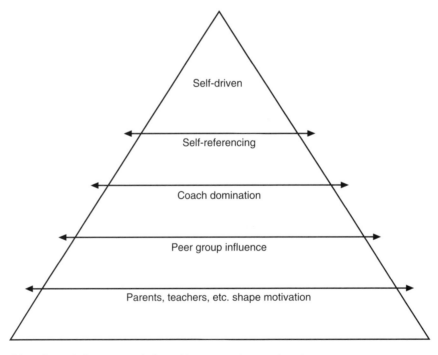

(Mentally weak dropouts are indicated by arrows at every stage.)

FIGURE 7.2   The route to self-motivation and mental toughness.

## Spinning Plates

Brent Erwin, head coach of women's soccer at Southern Methodist University in Dallas, once asked me to discuss mental toughness with his team. The women described their multiagenda personal program as spinning plates—with a chance at any moment that one will crash to the floor and break. They outlined their plates this way:

- Going to class and getting a degree
- Dealing with home and parents
- Building new and worthwhile relationships
- Living right off the field and staying healthy
- Attending practice
- Competing 100 percent in games
- Being at their best every day
- Doing their job for the team
- Being a good team member

These were all important issues for the women, and all of them had to be in harmony—no breakage—if they were to build focus and confidence. Coaches of women players should take note that women reevaluate their agendas on a daily basis, and problems will most likely affect practice unless coaches learn to observe performance changes and then identify strategies to help.

### Step 3: Establish a Work Ethic

For a player to feel positive and confident about the challenge of a tough match, he must feel physically capable of meeting the expected demands. Any questions about fitness, strength, and energy potential will begin to sow the seeds of doubt and anxiety, undermining performance before the player steps on the pitch. This may be a significant issue for these types of players:

- The young player in his debut
- The older player near the end of a career
- The player returning from injury
- The player faced with too many matches and insufficient recovery
- The player with poor nutrition
- The player with a damaging lifestyle
- The player playing out of position
- The player who has been asked to play too long or too often and has simply burned out

Motivation and confidence are inextricably linked with the willingness and capacity to work hard to ensure the best chance of success. When coaches and players work hard to prepare for a match, they build a belief that they have paid the price for victory. By committing to the effort, they become not only physically tougher but also mentally tougher.

Players, especially younger players, should read the autobiographies of former great players, in soccer and in other sports. They will find again and again the message of the importance of having a good work ethic. Julius Erving, the legendary Dr. J of basketball, says that it took him a whole career to be an overnight success. Golfer Nick Price emphasizes that it took him the whole of the 1980s to become an accomplished player in the 1990s.

Mentally tough players are the product not only of hard work but also smart work. They know when to work hard and when to recover. Within their training and lifestyle, they will incorporate good diet and nutrition, sufficient sleep, relaxation, and massage. Their self-discipline will always triumph over temptation; alcohol, drugs, and tobacco will not disrupt or harm their development. They do not see sport as a sacrifice but choose to live an athlete's life every day.

This book emphasizes that mental development can take place alongside physical development, so the smart player and coach will create a training program that allows for both. Intense practice should be based on whole-player excellence with drills that force players to work at high intensity while remaining mentally focused and making good decisions. When the going gets tough, the mentally tough player gets going!

## Step 4: Develop Self-Control

Being mentally tough means being positive in the face of adversity, especially when an occurrence in the match produces an emotional surge players may struggle to control. Loehr and McLaughlin (1990) identify the four responses the player may have when problems lead to emotional change.

- The player may tank, withdrawing energy and commitment.
- The player may become angry, directing energy negatively.
- The player may choke, becoming nervous and afraid.
- The player may respond to the challenge by investing additional positive energy to deal with the problem, the mentally tough way.

Mentally tough players see problems and setbacks as part of the territory if they wish to compete in soccer. When setbacks occur, they have the self-belief to view them as challenges to overcome. The player cannot choose what happens, but he can choose how to respond.

There is an excellent television advertisement in which the basketball great, Michael Jordan, details all the many failures in his career, including missing 22 end-of-game shots that decided the game. The message, of course, is that great players overcome the failures they suffer and always respond positively.

Dealing with criticism, mistakes, and victory or defeat is essential to a player's development. Therefore, much of my work is preparing players for likely scenarios through discussion and film, and then reviewing the potential actions. The players and I would examine examples of tanking, loss of temper, and choking before agreeing that exercising the self-control to meet the challenge is the best answer. The real tough guy is not the one who lashes out and loses control but the one who keeps control and walks away—the opposite of the common belief!

# Coaching for Mental Toughness

The attitude and behavior of the coach strongly influences the performance of the players. Coaches cannot expect to have a mentally tough team unless they both model and plan a program that emphasizes and reinforces positive winning attitudes.

## The Coach as a Role Model

The coach is an important and influential authority figure in players' lives. The body language, attitude, and expressions of the coach can shape, reinforce, or damage the players' self-esteem and confidence. This is especially true for younger players in a society with increasing numbers of one-parent families. The youth soccer coach, as a significant influence in a young person's life, often nowadays has a social responsibility as well as a coaching role.

If mental toughness is about meeting challenges with positive self-control, then the starting point, both in practice and competition, must be the coach. The coach must model every day those attitudes and behaviors that influence players toward a state of mental toughness. Never is the coach more tested than after a defeat. As Coach Parcells explains, "A coach lives in a black and white world—you win or you lose—and the black side stays with you longer" (1995, 3). The aftermath of defeat is a tough moment for a coach. She can choose to yell or sell, but the coach who wants a mentally tough team must demonstrate a controlled way to deal with emotional setbacks despite personal feelings. The coach must demonstrate an unshakeable perseverance and conviction towards the team's goals despite pressure or adversity.

The coach will find that a disciplined post-match routine is helpful in ensuring that she does not get either too high or too low. Many follow the 24 hour rule for staff and players: win or lose, it is time to move on after one day.

## Winning After Winning—
## A True Test of Mental Toughness

When the Norwegian club Stabaek FC faced a mentally demanding end-of-season situation, they called me in to advise. Lars Bohinen, the director of football, explained that with eight games to go, the team led the league and had reached the cup semi-final. The problem was that the previous season they had been in exactly the same situation—and collapsed.

Staying ahead of the pack in the final phase of the season is very much a challenge for mental toughness with three main essentials:

1. Champions define the situation; they don't let others define it for them.
2. Champions treat a pressure situation as an opportunity to succeed, not as an opportunity to fail.
3. The higher the stakes, the tougher the competition, the more daring you must be to carry the day.

With these points in mind, my advice to the players of Stabaek focused on the following:

● Remember why—achieving the dream is possible.
● Raise your bar—be at your best in this last part of the season.
● Stay positive—optimistic people achieve more.
● Trust yourself—believe in your ability and experience.
● Focus on performance—let results take care of themselves.
● Know your job—be clear on your role and responsibilities.
● Thrive on pressure—trust yourself to deliver.
● Stay cool—a loss is just an opportunity missed.
● Avoid distractions—match your lifestyle to your soccer.
● Stick to your routines—know your best preparation to play.
● Relax and enjoy—be intense without being tense.

Stabaek went on to win the league, celebrated, relaxed, then lost focus and lost the Cup final. Winning after winning is never easy!

### Creating the Mind-Set

Jim Thompson (1995), who has led the *Positive Coaching* movement in U.S. youth sports, neatly describes the impact of the coach on the team's mind-set and performance:

● Achievement needs energy,
● energy comes from emotions,

- emotions are released by ideas, and
- ideas come from coaches.

The successful coach will use ideas, stories, metaphors, films, and so on to shape the collective mind-set of the team and prepare them to be mentally tough in performance. If the coach shows an unwavering belief in the team's ability to achieve despite the obstacles, then the team has a framework for building the same mind-set and will become increasingly motivated.

Coaches can create a tough team mind-set by doing the following:

- Recruit tough character as well as talent.
- Find team leaders to drive the team on.
- Encourage the challenge within a team for selection and status.
- Set individual targets for players to reach.
- Create competitive hurdles, using competition to challenge the players every day.
- Ask tough questions in practices, and raise the bar
  - physically,
  - technically,
  - tactically,
  - mentally, and
  - emotionally.
- 'Buy' players competitive experience—players can't become mentally tough if they have not been through the fire of real competition sufficiently to deal with it.
- Give players nonstop feedback but stress accountability.
- Insist on player self-discipline.
- Help players make tough choices by teaching lifestyle skills and attitude.

## Learning Through Failure

Handling mistakes and failure is another area of responsibility for the coach. The coach's reaction to failure is key to the players' motivation and desire to work hard to correct mistakes. The coach has two choices:

- Use failure as an opportunity to give the players feedback on how to improve, and persuade them to recommit themselves to the effort with renewed motivation.
- Use failure as evidence of the players' inadequacy and proof that they cannot meet expectations. This emotional overreaction will demotivate the players.

Alan Goldberg, an experienced U.S. sport psychologist, explains why coaches must avoid the second option:

> The very worst thing a coach can teach an athlete is that mistakes and failing are bad and cause for humiliation. Punish or humiliate your athletes when they mess up and you will not only turn them into self-conscious, overly cautious underachievers, but you will also make them lose all respect for you. (1997, 70)

Soccer is learned through trial and error, and whatever the situation, mistakes will be made by both players and coaches. There may be very little difference in the number of mistakes that successful and unsuccessful players and coaches make; the difference is that the successful ones learn from their mistakes, recover well, and move on faster.

So important is this ability to recover from setbacks that Goldberg also adds:

> The feelings of failure are in reality the doorway to ultimate success..... of all the physical and mental qualities a player may possess, mental toughness is the most important. (70)

I particularly like the attitude of Wade Phillips, coach of the Dallas Cowboys, when he says to his team, "You take the responsibility for effort, and I'll take the responsibility for mistakes."

## Preparing Emotionally

Mental toughness begins with disciplined thinking under pressure followed by disciplined action. Coaches prepare players during practice to do the right things at the right time, combining thought and action.

The difference between practice and games is one of pressure and emotion; there are greater expectations and consequences in a game situation. Nothing can destroy a player's disciplined thinking more than the intervention of emotion—a sudden feeling of anxiety, helplessness, panic or even, as is so often the case, guilt and anger. A player at the mercy of emotion is out of control and rather than dealing in a prepared and thoughtful way with the situation, reacts in a negative and usually harmful manner. This is usually the case when a player is sent from the field. Coaches must prepare their players for the threat of emotional loss of control within the emotional roller coaster of a game in the following ways:

- Model personal composure in pressure situations.
- Make it clear that uncontrolled passion is the way to defeat. As I have stressed before, "Mental toughness is coming off the field with 11 players having won the game."

- Create simulated game conditions in practice, and insist on emotional control.
- Discuss with players (I always use film examples) the kind of "what if" scenarios that lead to the breakdown of disciplined thinking.
- Help players (a sport psychologist is useful here) learn to recognise and cope with a sudden burst of emotion and channel it positively back into the game (check the "traffic lights" example given in chapter 4).
- Teach the team to support each other when under pressure.
- Do not overcoach players: too much information creates anxiety and vulnerability on the field.
- Do not overtrain players: fatigue is the greatest destroyer of disciplined thought and action.

By controlling the mood of the players at training, often under exacting conditions, the coach is preparing the players emotionally for competition. When the pressure comes, the players then have a bank of responses and are not surprised and caught off-balance.

## Self-Referencing

One way that players become mentally tough is by accepting responsibility for their thoughts, feelings, and actions, and rejecting all possible excuses. Coaches can help by questioning and listening—not always telling players what they did wrong but encouraging them to talk about what they could have done better.

Perhaps the most complete basketball player ever, Michael Jordan was strong on this aspect of mental toughness.

> Players always want to blame someone else or some circumstance out of their control for their problems. You find a way not to accept the blame. The better players learn to say, "I played bad, but tomorrow I'll play better." A lot of younger players are afraid to admit they have bad nights, but everybody has bad nights, and it's how you rebound from these bad nights that dictates what kind of player you are going to be!

The coach can play a part in this by always encouraging the player to self-reference. Instead of giving the player a definition of the situation, the coach can ask the player to explain his actions: "How do you feel you played?" or "Why do you feel you behaved that way?" In this way the player must think through and account for his actions—a vital part of the learning process. The coach might borrow a thought from Rudyard Kipling for the notice board: "We have 40 million reasons, but not a single excuse."

# Building Team Toughness

If a coach wants to begin the process of building team toughness, he can start with a classroom exercise that raises awareness and understanding.

Coaches should ask the team to do the following:

1. Define team toughness.
2. Define individual player toughness.
3. Discuss team toughness:
   - Who is the toughest team to play?
   - Why are they so tough?
4. Discuss our team's toughness.
   - How do our opponents describe our toughness?
   - What do we need to do to become tougher?
5. Discuss individual toughness.
   - Who is the toughest player you have faced?
   - What made him so tough?
6. Discuss individual toughness.
   - What would opponents say about your toughness?
   - What can you do to increase your toughness?

## Summary

- What did you learn about yourself and your team?
- What specific strategies to build toughness did we identify?
- What individual and team goals can we set?

For further information of such exercises, see *101 Team Building Activities* by Dale and Conant (2004).

# Summary

The journey to soccer excellence will challenge the player at every step of the way. As players make their way up through the competitive levels, they must determine every day whether they can cope physically, technically, tactically, mentally, and emotionally. My experiences indicate that at the highest levels of soccer the physical, technical, and tactical differences between players become more marginal, and the real difference is the mental toughness available to deal with increased pressure. Such pressure will challenge the player's

- level of self-belief,
- ability to self-discipline,
- desire to compete every day,
- ability to deal with the sideshow,
- strength to deal with expectations of others, and
- resilience to recover from mistakes and setbacks.

Such mental toughness is based on each player building a strong self-identity, maintaining a high level of intrinsic motivation, being willing to practice hard and long, and having the composure to be self-controlled under pressure. As always the coach is a key part of this process, both as a model of mentally tough behavior and as a teacher of those attitudes, habits, and coping strategies that build a player's mental toughness. The greatest test for the coach will be his own ability to handle mistakes and setbacks in a positive manner in front of his players. Mental toughness starts with the personality and attitudes of the individual player but is enhanced by a team culture that consistently reinforces the value of being positive in the face of adversity.

# CHAPTER 8

# Competitiveness: Becoming a Match-Day Warrior

What I have learned about myself is that I am an animal
when it comes to achievement and wanting success.
There is never enough success for me.

**Gary Player, golfer**

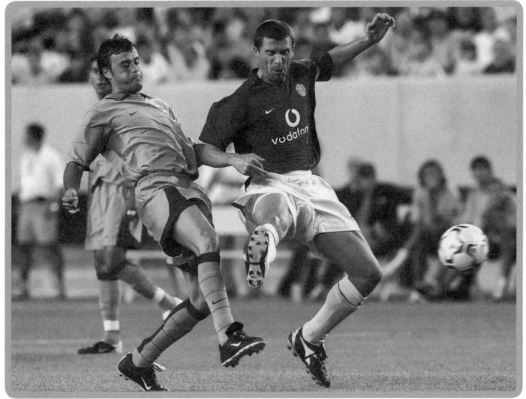

Andrew Budd/Action Images/Icon

O n my first day working at Manchester United I went out to observe practice. The top 16 players were working with Coach Steve McClaren on an 8v8 possession game. I was impressed with the quality and intensity and quickly realized that when a team gave up the ball, it could be some time, and a lot of hard defending, before they got it back.

At one point Dennis Irwin had the ball under pressure, and his teammate Roy Keane made a very intelligent run to get free for him. Despite Roy signaling clearly, Dennis didn't react and lost the ball. To my amazement, Roy Keane ran 40 yards to vent his anger directly to Irwin, "Get your ... head up!" Irwin apologized, but the intensity of the game clearly went up. When I mentioned this at the coaches meeting, two things emerged.

1. Such internal challenges were welcomed, and often made practice more challenging than games. One coach said, "We win Saturday matches on rainy Tuesday mornings."

2. Roy Keane was a true warrior-athlete whose competitive fire never dimmed and as a result always got the best out of himself and the players around him.

In all the profiles of great players and great teams, those with competitive fire, the need to challenge and win at every competitive opportunity, are always highlighted. Such players are always driven by strong intrinsic motivation, their emotional need for success feeding their need to compete and desire to win and be the best. This competitive fire leads to their special performance characteristics:

- Ability to respond to pressure
- Capacity to confront opposition aggressively
- Capacity for focused concentration
- Courage to deal with pain
- Consistent desire to improve
- Ability to learn, adapt—do what it takes to win
- Ability to play smart as well as hard

## I Can't Play Friendlies

Some seasons ago Manchester United won the league championship after defeating Southampton away from home. With five games still to go in the league program, this was a remarkable achievement and cause for great celebration at the end of the game. On the bus to the airport and the flight back to Manchester, Roy Keane quietly asked the coaches not to select him for the remaining five games. When asked why Roy said, "I can't play friendlies."

For an athlete who thrives on competitive fire, a game without meaning is an ordeal.

Soccer is a game of challenge, constantly testing both players' and coaches' ability to find their own competitive fire. The higher the levels, the more this will become an essential resource for success.

However, as I have stressed throughout this book, the major threat to a player's potential is himself—his doubts, anxieties, and fears getting in the way of his self-belief, confidence, and competitive fire. To be strong, each player must first of all overcome his performance anxiety.

# Beating Performance Anxiety

Comedian Woody Allen once said that 80 percent of success is just showing up. The starting point for soccer players is finding the courage to overcome the fears that the challenge of competition produces.

All players face performance anxiety (see the sidebar below), but the players who compete face up to their fears, overcome them, and convert them into positive energy. Coaches must teach their players by helping them frame positive answers for their internal dialogue. Coaches must be confidence-givers; all leaders must exude confidence: "If the bugle call is uncertain, then who will prepare for battle?" (1 Cor. 14:8).

When South Carolina women's soccer head coach, Shelley Smith, asked me to discuss performance anxiety with her large group of freshmen, I began by asking them to fill a flipchart full of the doubts, anxieties, and fears of being a freshman scholar-athlete. Once we had a page full of the negatives, I then asked them to provide the most positive response they could think of for each negative. We filled another page!

## PERFORMANCE ANXIETY

The key questions that a player's internal dialogue has to answer are the following:

- Do I want to do this?
- Do I believe I can do this today?
- What are the risks?
- How might the audience judge me?
- Can I deal with failure?
- Can I deal with success?
- What if the unexpected happens?
- Can I cope with the sideshow?
- What else could I be doing?

As a result

- the coaches now know the performance anxiety agenda,
- each athlete now has a stock of prepared positive answers to each likely instance of performance anxiety,
- the athletes know they are not alone in their fears, and
- the freshman group enjoyed the chance to share something together, and as a result, became closer.

## Journey to Competitiveness

Figure 8.1 illustrates the route that players must take if they wish to reach the highest level of competitive form—the state of flow. This journey represents a personal game plan for players, who should check their strengths or weaknesses with their coaches at each stage. The competition for places should mean that players who cannot deal with any particular stage of the journey will find themselves rejected.

Following are the key points for each stage.

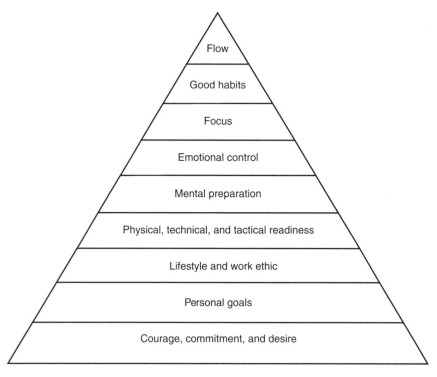

FIGURE 8.1   The route to the state of flow.

## Courage, Commitment, and Desire

The starting point for players who undertake this difficult journey is a dream that inspires and motivates them to face up to the challenge. Unless a player dreams of being the best, it is unlikely that she will find the motivation to overcome the hurdles along the way. Coaches must reinforce the dream for each player and the team at every opportunity and teach them to see challenges rather than problems.

## Personal Goals

The player lacking direction can waste energy and determination, so each player should spend time establishing personal goals, both long- and short-term. I sometimes stop players and ask them why they have to come to practice. They generally respond, "To improve." I then ask, "Improve what?" and so on. This sort of conversation helps players realize that practice is the best opportunity for working on their personal goals and reminds them why they need to make the effort.

Barrell and Ryback (2008), sport psychology consultants to leading U.S. professional teams, note that the most competitive and successful athletes focus on doable goals. They select a limited number of things that they can be exceptional at and focus solely on these.

## Lifestyle and Work Ethic

"You play how you live" is often quoted to young players. The greatest challenge they face may well be lifestyle issues. Lifestyle usually has its most dramatic effect on a player's work ethic. I once heard Dan O'Brien, Olympic decathlon champion, respond to the question asking how he became the champion. He wrote two numbers on the board—1,500 and 36—and then explained that it took him 1,500 hours of training to prepare for 36 minutes of explosive activity on the track. O'Brien knows that only

## Competitive Gold

On their return from the Beijing Olympics, I watched the British gold medal winners being interviewed. Especially interesting was the competitive mind-set of the young female cyclist, Nicole Cooke.

When reminded of her four-year chase for a gold medal, she replied she had never chased a gold medal. Rather, she had done the right thing every day and let the gold medal come to her. When reminded of the sacrifices she had made, she replied she had made no sacrifices whatsoever—but had made a lot of good choices. Being competitive is a state of mind where there are no excuses.

in the dictionary does success come before work and that living a healthy lifestyle is the only way to manage such a workload and stay competitive every day.

## Physical, Technical, and Tactical Readiness

We cannot compete if we are fatigued, if we cannot control the ball, or if we are confused about tactical decisions. Fundamental preparation, often more about perspiration than inspiration, underpins success. To achieve competitive excellence, players must know that they can do their job physically, technically, and tactically. Bill Walsh made this a priority as he turned the San Francisco 49ers from losers to Super Bowl champions:

> Our coaching staff was meticulous and tenacious in analyzing and then teaching the requirements of each player's position. They then created multiple drills for each one of those individual skills, which were then practiced relentlessly until their execution at the highest level was automatic—routine perfection. (2009, 17-18)

## Mental Preparation

Once they have made the commitment and worked hard to prepare physically and technically, players have begun to build a winning attitude. From good preparation should come a strong sense of self-identity, confidence, and the foundations of mental toughness. Obstacles and setbacks will inevitably delay progress, so success may well depend on the player's ability to stay mentally positive and resilient. The truly competitive player may appear very selfish, focusing on his job and finding a way for his team to win while appearing insensitive and unyielding to any other concerns.

## Emotional Control

Having created the right frame of mind and a competitive attitude, players must establish a personal strategy to maintain it under game pressure. Physically, the player may be well prepared to compete, but games take place in an emotional context. The discipline of emotional control is essential to preventing the mind from getting in the way of the body. The warrior-athlete is characterized by the passion to win, but passion without control can render a player vulnerable. Self-discipline and self-management are key qualities.

## Focus

To play throughout a game at a highly competitive level, players need to build their capacity for focused concentration. A loss of focus for one moment is all it takes to lose a game. The ability to maintain a state of concentration is a critical factor in competitiveness. When Barrell and Ryback studied factors that predicted future athletic success they concluded, "the single most important factor was an ability to stay present to what was going on and not get 'sucked in' by negativity or pressure" (2008, 85).

Players must learn the warning signs that indicate they are focusing on themselves instead of the situation. Applying intense focus expends a great amount of energy. Mentally tough players understand the need for proper recovery and relaxation: they come to each game with their batteries recharged. When Dan O'Brien was asked about the most important skill he had learned, he replied that it was the skill of forgetting, or letting go. He emphasized the importance of being able to clear the mind after being involved in one piece of action, especially one with a negative result, in order to be focused, positive, and relaxed for the next.

### Good Habits

The state of flow is often described as a no-think situation in which the body works automatically. Trust is an important ingredient. Players will perform best if they get their minds—and possible doubts and anxieties—out of the way and trust the habits they have programmed into their bodies. I work every week with players who survive important games not on new behavior they suddenly create but on good habits established over many years of work. Train and trust!

Thus the journey to competitiveness and flow calls for a great deal of responsibility on the part of the player. But that's what separates the great players from the rest. Here, too, players can learn much by reading accounts of the great players in all sports, not only soccer. For example, Halberstam's (1999) wonderful analysis of Michael Jordan's career illustrates many aspects of competitiveness and shows how Michael became the most competitive team player in the world—playing in the flow night after night.

## Competitiveness at Practice

The desire and drive to be at our best and win is a habit that must be present every time there is challenge. Practice is the breeding ground of such habits, and it is here the players and coaches must work to build competitive fire. There are, of course, players who feel they can simply switch competitiveness on when game time arrives, but my experience is that players who find reasons to go easy in practice will find reasons to go easy in games.

Coaches need to find ways to create intensity in practice while managing energy and injuries. All the coaches I have worked alongside would prefer a shorter, more intense, and challenging practice than a longer, more

## Competitive Fire Overcomes Performance Anxiety

After Roy Keane I would select Jamie Carragher, Liverpool's centerback, as the player who most demonstrates competitive fire—dominance and consistency every day. In his autobiography, *Carra*, Jamie gives a player's view of performance anxiety when coming off at halftime 3-0 down in the 2005 European Cup final.

> *As I walked towards the dressing room, I was suffering from a depressing combination of despondency and humiliation. I couldn't bear to lift my head up and glimpse the faces in the crowd, or the banners and red jerseys scattered around the stadium. I looked towards the floor and saw nothing but endless dejection. My dreams had turned to dust; I wasn't thinking about the game anymore. My thoughts were with my family and friends. I was so sorry. . . . There was a sense of shame to go with my sorrow. The Liverpool fans had taken over the stadium, and there was nothing we could do to make amends. I almost began to regret reaching The Final. (2008, 271)*

Despite this Jamie's good competitive habits came to the fore in the second half as Liverpool turned the game around to tie the game at 3-3 and then win the penalty shoot-out—a true test of competitive toughness.

> *Courage, character, grit, willpower and raw strength—these are the virtues people have instilled in me since I was seven years old. I'd come a long way from the snotty-nosed kid who wanted to come off the pitch early because it was raining. I bet if there is one moment my dad rewinds on DVD, it's that one. (278)*

Jamie refers to the first challenge to his competitive fire when he was 7 years old and wanted to stop playing because of the rain—but together he, his parents, and his coaches overcame this challenge and the many that followed, developing a competitiveness that has led Jamie to the highest honors.

relaxed session. Even on light training days, there is a case for an 8- or 12-minute period of high intensity where coaches can teach their players to compete at game intensity. This is particularly true for female players who might find competitiveness and intensity uncomfortable. Matina Horner, in DeBoer, explains this:

> Women appeared to have a problem with competitive achievement. . . . This fear exists because for most women, the anticipation of success in competitive achievement activity produces anticipation of certain negative consequences—for example, threat of social rejection and loss of femininity. (2004, 52)

With a basis of good relationships and trust in the group, the coach must urge them to build a competitive mind-set where they accept it is okay to compete, be a leader, stand out, and so on. Players who wish to increase competitiveness should do the following:

- Recognize practice as the key to improvement.
- Set personal targets for every practice.
- Come to practice clear of other life issues.
- Be first on the field.
- Quit socializing once the white line is crossed.
- Visualize themselves as great competitors.
- Be first to every drill, huddle, and so on.
- Stay focused on every action taken.
- Think like a winner, feel like a winner, and act like a winner.
- Enjoy success and forget mistakes.
- Urge teammates to be more competitive.
- Be last off the field.

# Pregame Competitiveness

I always remind players that pregame starts much earlier than their arrival in the dressing room. It is their responsibility to arrive at the game well rested, with a clear mind free of potential distractions. When Middlesbrough won the Carling Cup on a Sunday, we had devoted the previous Monday and Tuesday to administration and media. From Wednesday onward, nothing was allowed but a focus on soccer.

Each player must build a pregame performance routine that ensures the best mental and emotional state to start the game. Players differ in style and routine of preparation. Areas must be found in the dressing room for the introvert, who will prefer space and privacy, and the extrovert, who can follow a routine while happily interacting with others. Although styles will vary, each player must have a routine that clears the mind and allows focus only on soccer issues. Each player must build a pregame competitive state by doing the following:

- Thinking and acting in a totally positive manner
- Ignoring any negatives such as moaners
- Talking themselves up and focusing on the success that got them to this point
- Getting control of their emotions and maintaining perspective and practicing relaxation
- Building arousal using inspirational material
- Slowly narrowing focus and increasing intensity
- Reviewing constantly the three most important things they will do to contribute to their team's success

Players must accomplish all this while being relaxed and enjoying the moment. Of course, experience is a major factor in developing sound pregame coping strategies.

Coaches can help by trying various ways to influence the mental state of their players in the dressing room—motivational talks, humor, video, music, wall posters, cue cards, and so on.

## Competitiveness in the Game

As General Colin Powell once said, "No battle plan survives contact with the enemy." A team may occasionally maintain the pregame state of mind for the whole 90 minutes, but the opponent will usually produce difficult and unsettling moments. The player must now reveal mental toughness by thriving on the pressure.

The bottom line is control—the player must first exert self-control and then exercise control over the opponents and the game situations he is involved in. As we have emphasized, in the heat of the game the player relies on these physical and mental habits:

- Maintaining an unwavering self-belief
- Having a winning attitude (exemplified by the player who commits for the full 90 minutes, never losing but simply running out of time)
- Focusing only on what he can control
- Having the discipline to do the job
- Managing anger and mistakes
- Being able to forget the bad moments and having the resilience to bounce back
- Having the courage to take a risk when the situation demands it
- Enjoying the satisfaction of competition

## Remaining Competitive at Halftime

After 45 minutes comes a wonderful period that allows players to absorb the lessons of the first half and recompose their mental and emotional state in preparation for the second half. Players should develop a miniroutine to stay focused despite the sometimes overemotional atmosphere engendered by coaches. Great teams and great players use halftime as a springboard for even greater efforts, reviewing both physical and mental determination. As American football coach Woody Hayes said,

> The only thing compulsory for my team is that we are at our strongest in the final quarter.

## Win the Second Half

While at Middlesbrough FC, I assisted Paul Barron, our excellent goalkeeping coach, at an away game at Manchester United with our very young, but potentially good, second team. Paul and I enjoyed the chance to prepare this group of youngsters for a difficult challenge and started the game with high hopes.

At halftime we came in 2-0 down, but Paul and I took the time to reflect before we came up with the halftime message. Our view was that we were playing well despite conceding two unfortunate goals. The players were clearly down, but Paul and I gave them a very uplifting halftime where we expressed our disappointment at the goals conceded and the chances missed but quickly moved on to emphasize our delight at some of the good soccer we had played. We then set them the challenge: Win the second half!

Teams stay competitive when they see a target they can achieve. A team losing at halftime might see that target fading away, and it is the job of the coach to renew that target or find a new one to inspire their team's competitiveness. Never let your team give up on a game before the final whistle!

Our team of youngsters went back on the field ready to meet a new challenge, worked hard, found their form, and won 3-2. Paul and I rewarded them in the time-honored British fashion of buying them all fish and chips on the way home.

## Dealing With the Postgame

We recognize the postgame as a time for physical cool-down, but we may not use it effectively for mental and emotional calming. Players and coaches must handle victory or defeat in a way that provides for evaluation and learning but does not damage a player's self-belief or self-esteem, which could produce future fear instead of confidence. Players must find a way of dealing with the postgame passion and moving on to a calm perspective of their performance—a personal evaluation. When they have dealt with the formalities and found their space, they might ask themselves these questions:

- How do I feel about today?
- What did I learn?
- Did I achieve my personal goals?
- What obstacles stood in my way?
- Did I get in the way of my own performance?
- Do I need a discussion with the coach or sport psychologist?

- Do I need to amend my routines for pregame and halftime?
- What is my personal action plan to prepare for the next game?

Whatever the postgame strategy, the most important point is that it ends with the player looking forward to the next game.

# Summary

I have had the good fortune to work with many great players, and the one characteristic that has impressed me the most has been their competitiveness. Both Roy Keane and Jamie Carragher, the two players I refer to in this chapter, are good people off the field but, because of their desire, become competitive warriors when they cross the white line.

That is not to say that neither experiences doubt or fear. Every player faces performance anxiety but, with the help of empathic coaches, has to learn to overcome it and build competitive toughness—a "play anywhere, play anytime, play anybody" streak of steely determination.

Although the journey to competitive toughness starts with the personality of the player and the impact of their parents, the coach has great teaching opportunities during practice and games. It is important that from an early age coaches, within the context of age, gender, and level, set competitive hurdles that challenge their players every time they come to practice.

Being competitive is a state of mind—the body merely follows instructions—and so players are reminded of the importance of pregame preparation. Actors warm up to their role before they go on stage, and so must soccer players.

The game itself, as well as halftime, will provide a constant test to the player and team's competitive toughness. Players and coaches are urged to maintain self-belief, deal with setbacks, focus on now, and never, ever quit on a game. Thus are the habits of competitiveness built. As Aristotle once stated, "Excellence is not an act but a habit."

# CHAPTER 9

# Communication: Sharing Information Effectively

Yelling doesn't communicate. It's a whisper in somebody's ear. It's a pat on the back. It's a push at times. Whatever you need to do to communicate. It's not jamming somebody up against the wall. It's learning what you can and cannot say to each individual to get the best out of them.

**Mo Vaughn, baseball player**

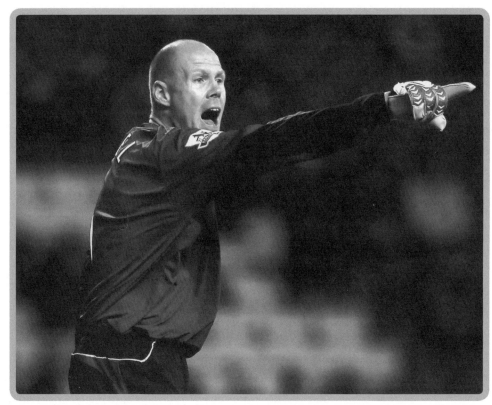

One of the elements of changing a soccer club from a losing culture to a winning culture is communication. A characteristic of losing teams is a decline in the amount and quality of communication. Thus, when Steve McClaren and I were appointed at Middlesbrough FC and found a losing culture, improving communication became a priority. These were our strategies:

- Daily coaching staff meetings
- Weekly team meetings
- Weekly unit meetings—goalkeeping, defense, attack
- Monthly all-staff meetings, including noncoaching support staff
- Daily updated communication via whiteboards
- Informal contact in the corridors
- Delegating me as a neutral listener, always available to all
- Delegating Steve Harrison, a well-loved senior coach, as the dressing room coach to pick up the mood of the players
- Senior group meetings—an occasional get-together with our senior players
- A weekly meeting with the captain

Over time, improved relationships were established through good communication and reflected our policy of relating to players rather than handling them. Slowly the culture changed, self-belief and confidence grew, and a winning culture emerged. Increase communication; decrease anxiety!

If this book helps to develop more complete players and coaches by involving them in the wider issues of mental, emotional, and lifestyle aspects of performance, then to a great extent, it will depend on extending the language of soccer and the ability of players and coaches to communicate effectively with these new terms.

Soccer has always had its own language covering physical and technical performance—the simple language of command and response. But soccer is increasingly more complex and sophisticated. Players are better educated and more independent. The coach today will have to deal with all of this to create a cohesive team that meets all challenges.

Communication, in all forms and modes, has begun an inexorable rise to the top of the agenda, and a coach or player without the ability to give and receive the information necessary for the highest levels of performance will suffer. Figures 9.1 and 9.2 (page 140) illustrate the demands placed on players and coaches to be effective communicators. They must be able to interact successfully with a variety of people in a range of styles and situations. The extended language of soccer by which players and coaches transmit their thoughts and feelings will involve several modes:

*Self-talk* Players should recognize the importance of disciplining the inner voice to stay positive.

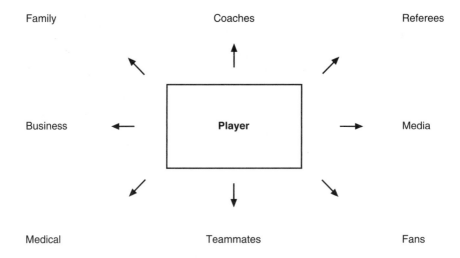

FIGURE 9.1 The player and communication.

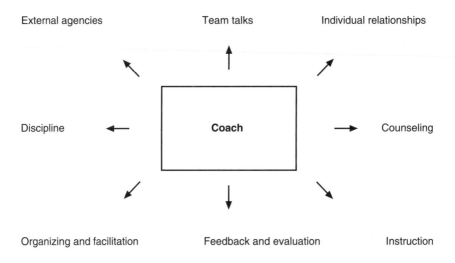

FIGURE 9.2 Responsibilities of a coach dependent on communication skill.

*Verbal* The majority of soccer interactions occur on the move, and verbal dexterity can be important to success.

*Listening* A major shift for coaches, and some players, will be recognizing the need to develop good listening skills.

*Connecting* Communicating beyond technical needs can build the personal relationships—coach–player bonds and player–player bonds—that build team chemistry.

*Body language*   It is not just what is said but also the way it is expressed that communicates the complete message. Coaches, in particular, must be careful that their body language does not betray them.

*Visual*   Most players can retain no more than three points that a coach might make orally. A list on a flip chart or a poster on the locker-room wall, however, might help players absorb more detail by allowing them to return to the message several times.

*Technological*   The modern player is accustomed to receiving messages sent technologically, and coaches must become familiar with these new opportunities—e-mails, texting, and so on—to stimulate and educate. University of Louisville basketball coach Rick Pitino is going even further.

> We're now exploring an intranet system that would allow me to send video clips of specific plays to the players, so they can quickly absorb lessons on what they did well and did not do well in that day's practice. A soon as practice is over, we can break it down on video in all aspects, with a heavy emphasis on execution and effort. . . . It saves us time instead of having to call them in the next day, and it allows them to judge for themselves how they did and where they can improve their performance. I believe it will help us in three ways: (1) It will provide immediate feedback, when the practice remains fresh in their heads; (2) It will ground them in the reality of what they did and did not do, as opposed to tricking themselves into thinking they performed better than they really did; and (3) It will motivate them to improve and give greater effort the next day. (2008, 191-192)

Clearly, the coach or player must communicate in a way that suits his personality and philosophy. But coaches and players should recognize that it is important to learn the skills required of all forms of communication. Such efforts can bring worthwhile rewards.

## Principles of Good Communication

No matter what the context, knowledge of the fundamental principles of communication are essential for both players and coaches:

- Know and use the other person's name. This is both courteous and relaxing.
- Be prepared by knowing what you want the outcome to be.
- Be empathic. Try to understand the viewpoint of the other person. The goal is to connect, not to defeat.
- Be relaxed and open; avoid negative body language.
- Face the person you are talking to and establish eye contact.

- Choose a style according to the person you are talking to. Simple is usually best.
- Remain on the agenda; don't become sidetracked.
- Be objective and control emotions.
- Be honest. Don't say one thing and mean another.
- Occasionally seek clarification that your message has been received and understood.
- Repeat key messages. Find alternate ways to emphasize them.
- Lighten things up whenever possible with a little humor.
- Allow time for questions.
- Listen attentively using good body language.
- Try to understand and make allowance for different cultures.
- In concluding the conversation, try to sum up what has been agreed on.
- Set an agreed to action plan for future behavior.

# Breakdown in Communication

By understanding the barriers to communication, coaches and players may be able to prevent some of them from being erected. Listed here are typical barriers I have seen that impeded the communication process:

*Assumptions*   Coaches assume players know what is required of them, and players assume that coaches know how they (the players) feel.

*Differences of opinion*   Although unavoidable, differences must lead to more communication, not less. Parties should agree to disagree.

*Personality clashes*   This, too, is inevitable, but with communication, a common ground can be established so that personal issues can be put aside for team needs.

*Role conflicts*   Players will resent playing roles that do not fit their perception of their best contribution, but coaches can ease matters by sharing their reasons. Perhaps a consensus can be reached. Uncertainty of roles and expectations will create a defensive climate within a team.

*Power struggles*   Teams are always evolving, and the pecking order will always be considered important. Unless the head coach or team captain settles this by clear and shared communication, matters will only deteriorate.

*Cultural misunderstandings*   Great care must be taken to recognize and understand culturally influenced communication. Coaches must consider the words they use and their body language in expressing their message. They should always check that the players are clear about what they, the coaches, have said.

## CRITICIZING A PLAYER

Coaches must give players feedback and make them accountable without damaging relationships. This can easily go wrong if the following guidelines are ignored:

- Try to criticize in private.
- Do not speak until the player is emotionally ready to listen.
- Do not speak if you are out of control.
- Focus on the behavior, not the person.
- Begin by pointing out some of the good things the player is doing.
- State clearly what the problem is; be specific.
- State clearly what the correct behavior should be; be specific.
- Check that the player understands.
- Ask the player for his view.
- Show understanding for the player's situation.
- Ask the player if he wants to change.
- Ask the player how he can change.
- Agree to an action plan.

*Perceived injustices*   Soccer often requires instant decision making, producing many opportunities for conflict. Coaches must always have the power to make such decisions, and the players must have the discipline to carry them out. At the same time, it is beneficial to have in place a feedback process that releases tension rather than builds it.

*Role changes*   Events occur every day in professional clubs (nonselection, injury, loss of form) that force players into role changes and possible loss of status. A rapid decline in communication often follows, thereby exacerbating the problem. Coaches and players must be sensitive to this and find ways of maintaining supportive communication.

## Creating a Communication Network

Whenever I have worked in a turnaround situation, my major contribution has been in moving the club from a defensive climate of communication—cliques, power struggles, detachment of some individuals from the group, personal attacks instead of performance criticism—to a supportive climate with positive communication and a shared ownership of the issues facing the team. Within soccer teams, the quantity and quality of interaction will always fluctuate as team membership changes, presenting new faces and new personalities, but certain measures help accommodate the shifts and maintain a positive climate:

*Honesty*   Always try for clear, consistent, direct communication that is honest and contains no hidden agendas. The criterion is that if it's what is best for the team, there is no problem sharing it. One of the differences I have found between assistant coaches and head coaches is that although both can communicate good news, it is the head coach who has the strength and personality to deliver bad news.

*Feedback*   Players need constant feedback. Players do not get enough regular feedback on their performance and progress. Coaches should be feedback machines and spend a great deal of time preparing instructions and comments for the players.

*Stability*   Too many changes can upset the mental and emotional stability of the team, increasing anxiety and decreasing communication. Coaches should have constant discussions about the benefit of stability against the advantage of change.

*Continuity of selection*   Being on the team is important for every player. Generally, a squad of players comes to terms with who is likely to be on the team and who is not. Although change will always occur, a high level of continuity is key to maintaining positive attitudes and communication, and therefore, performance.

*Core and fringe*   Every team is likely to have core players (continuous selections who carry much of the responsibility) and fringe players who are not yet regulars. The head coach will see core players regularly as a group and the captain once every week. This provides opportunities for early warning signals and helps the coach understand the mood of the dressing room and avoid conflict.

*Team talks*   These are extremely valuable in communicating information to everybody efficiently and effectively. For a coach with good communication skills, such talks can be a very powerful tool to shape both the motivation and the emotional state of the team.

*Film*   The use of film, the most natural form of communication for some of our modern players, has increased dramatically. Teams can now more easily create their own film clips and target them for motivational or educational purposes. It is often true that a key image has more impact than a thousand words.

*Focus groups*   For particular issues, for example, the play of the goalkeeper and the back four defenders, the coaches will not hesitate to meet with only the players concerned, holding a discussion supported by film evidence. Similarly, I may conduct a team-building exercise in which we

## The Five-Minute Team Talk

Coaches need to be reminded that players often don't see the big picture and thus lose track of purpose and progress. This was true of a women's soccer team I was advising, so I asked the coach if I could conduct a five-minute meeting on the field at the start of practice. The coach agreed and gathered the women around the center circle. The meeting went something like this:

- Q. "Just remind me where this team is going."
- A. The players restated the team's mission.
- Q. "Where are we now?"
- A. The players explained progress to date.
- Q. "So what do we have to do today?"
- A. The players emphasized the importance of practice.
- Q. "So how can *you* help today?"
- A. Each athlete agreed to be at her best.
- "So let's go."
- The players whooped and dashed to the first practice.

This kind of meeting can be held in less than five minutes but is valuable for putting a team back on track with its purpose and progress—as well as for reinvigorating attitude.

agree on our team goals for the next season. Such agreements will form the basis for further discussion during the season.

*One-on-one*   At the end of the day, soccer is a personal challenge. The most important communication in a club is the one-on-one discussions between coach and coach, coach and player, and player and player. These need not be formalized; players often feel more comfortable when they happen in an informal context. Coaches must seek these contact moments, taking care to talk to all players, not just the stars. Some coaches record such interactions to ensure that they do not ignore anyone for too long. I have found this to be the best way of learning the needs, hopes, and goals of each player.

## Communication and the Player

Soccer is a team game played in a social setting. No player can remain isolated from the variety of external pressures to communicate. As always with pressure, the player has the choice of avoiding challenge, coping with it, or thriving on it. Rick Pitino is clear that players have no choice because if they can't communicate, they won't be successful. He goes on to say that those who can communicate will benefit:

> Communication is about making contact with others who can help you achieve your goals—and you in turn can help them achieve theirs. Even though you are on the road to self-improvement, it's not a journey you are taking in a vacuum. (1997, 118)

As players reach higher levels, the problems that can destroy progress—nonselection, injury, loss of form, change of clubs, personal and family problems, and so on—become more significant. Communication is the only way to start solving these problems. The player needs to have the cour-

## Communication Ice Breaker

For teams assembled with players from different clubs or teams that have recruited several new players, I have a favorite ice-breaking game that encourages shared communication in a nonthreatening and enjoyable way.

The players all sit in a circle, and the captain holds a ball. I inform them that on a flip chart I have written several questions, each on a separate page, that I want them to answer. The captain starts by answering the first question. After answering, he throws the ball to someone else in the circle, who repeats the process. Each question will be shown for only three minutes, and then I will flip over to the next question.

The trick is to start with nonthreatening questions and then slowly move the team to issues I really want them to debate. Here are the questions I used when working with a women's soccer team that had some team cohesion problems:

Q1. The best thing about playing soccer is . . .

Q2. The worst thing about playing soccer is . . .

Q3. The team I admire most is . . . because . . .

Q4. The team that disappoints me most is . . . because . . .

Q5. The player I admire most is . . . because . . .

Q6. The player who disappoints me most is . . . because . . .

Q7. The teammate I admire most is . . . because . . .

Q8. The three key things I can offer this team are . . .

Q9. This team would do better if . . .

In this simple half-hour exercise, the questions can be varied to focus the communication on the team's specific problems. In such a fast-moving exercise, a high degree of honesty and disclosure often occurs, and the coach should have a relevant agenda to follow up on.

age and confidence to seek help. My role with teams is to ensure that no player becomes isolated, and I am often the first point of contact. Players may wish to follow these guidelines:

- Build a positive support group of people they know they can go to who will listen and help.
- Listen and learn from criticism; accept it as part of developing excellence.
- Be open with teammates and become part of a supportive network of communication. One characteristic of successful teams is that players are willing to challenge each other to perform better. David Whitaker, former Great Britain field hockey coach, agrees: "Players in a strong team can often take harsher words from one another than they can take from management" (1999, 90).
- When teams can deal with this, they raise the level of internal challenge and therefore, performance. However, I do advise players to challenge in positive ways. A player who has made a bad pass will respond better to "Come on, you're better than that" rather than direct criticism, which may shake his confidence even further.
- Develop good listening powers; be open to learning from everyone.
- Learn to maintain communication in emotional situations.
  - Cope with the give and take of the club.
  - Deal with the difficult issues in an open, straightforward way.
  - Share information.
  - Accept the bad news as readily as the good.

## Communication and the Team

When a sport psychologist investigates problems within a team, he searches for hot spots through questioning and observation. In most cases, the hot spots are communication problems. Typical problem situations include the following:

- Conflict being managed badly
- Cultural differences, especially with the talented Afro-Caribbean and South American players
- Coach intimidation
- The coach not listening, so players feel their problems are not being dealt with
- Channels of communication being mixed up.

Some tension and anxiety is inevitable in a team striving to achieve, but the only way to relieve this is to increase communication and the feeling of shared ownership of the problems.

Chapter 11 examines the building of team cohesion and the role of effective and regular communication. Table 9.1 highlights this by emphasizing the communication elements necessary for both coach and players in building team chemistry. In each step of the team-building process, the communication responsibilities for coaches and players are identified.

| TABLE 9.1—Communication for Building Team Chemistry | | |
|---|---|---|
| **The coach should** | **Intended effect on the team-building process (the action plan)** | **The player should** |
| Inspire | The coach sells the vision | Listen |
| Listen | Players buy into the vision | Commit |
| Discuss | Team's operating procedures and shared ownership agreed to in discussion | Discuss and question |
| Accept as role model | Team values and identity confirmed by consensus | Accept as role model |
| Clarify | Review the process so far | Understand |
| Challenge | Set team goals | Accept |
| Appreciate individuals | Set individual goals | Be open and assertive |
| Be positive | Hard work, support, encouragement | Be positive |
| Be constructive, not personal | Instruction, challenge, evaluation, and feedback | Listen attentively |
| Control emotions | Mistake management and correction | Understand and accept |
| Praise | Reward and reinforce good play | Enjoy |
| Conduct meetings | Maintain flow of information | Maintain awareness |
| Seek player enjoyment | Humor eases; worry prolongs | Contribute to enjoyment |
| Be open—fair but firm | Apply discipline when necessary | Accept and move on |
| Offer empathy | Deal with player's lifestyle problems | Seek help |
| Keep communicating | Handle the bad times | Keep communicating |
| Increase communication | Resolve conflicts | Increase communication |
| Listen and respect | Support player's individual needs at competition time | Be assertive to control situation |

# Communication and the Coach

Communication is the first step to success for every coach. As Bill Parcells puts it, "Coaching is an act of communication—of explaining what you want of people in a way that allows them to do it" (1995, 129).

In my observation of coaches, who are often ex-players working at the highest levels, I've identified three major communication issues:

**1.** Coaches allow their emotions to become involved when watching games. They become spectators rather than analytical observers. They fail to note some of the important points that might help their teams. Halftime, then, may become an expression of emotion rather than objective communication targeted on winning the game.

**2.** Coaches have little training in communication. Most do not use the power of the flip chart, match analysis data, or film, for example. One of the ways to avoid the boredom of repeating important messages is to vary the format. If the coach is talented technically but communicates poorly, it makes sense to use a skilled assistant or a sport psychologist to take the lead occasionally in team talks or individual counseling.

**3.** Coaches often become so wrapped up in the process of teaching soccer that they forget that people are involved. An example of such ineffective communication was quoted in the *Football Coaches Association Journal* in which Leif Isberg (1997) monitored the instructions that youth coaches gave to players. In three matches, coaches sent 116, 187, and 55 messages to players to change behavior. Isberg classified 67, 55, and 12 of those totals as ineffective because the coaches failed to use a player's name, producing uncertainty. The following sidebar encourages coaches to empathize with their players better by showing the key questions every player needs to have answered.

Some useful guidelines for coaches include the following:

- All communication from the coach is important, so be sure that players cannot misinterpret your messages.
- Be proactive and communicate when you see a problem. Don't wait and hope it will go away.
- Use positive language that creates positive expectancies of the players. Challenge the players to be better rather than punishing them for being poor.
- Never assume.
- Make every communication seem important. Show respect to all players.
- Allow time for everybody. Research indicates that coaches spend far more time (up to seven times more!) with star players.

- Never promise anything you cannot deliver.
- Never threaten anything you cannot enforce.
- Be aware of body language when communicating. Lombardi (1996) reports a fascinating study by Mehrabian, who examined factors influencing coach-to-player communication. Only 7 percent of the impact was derived from the verbal message (the words used); 38 percent of the impact emerged from the vocal (how the words were said), and 55 percent of the impact depended on the nonverbal (the body language used).
- In order to reinforce players' self-esteem, balance praise with criticism (the sandwich technique is praise-criticism-praise). Tip the balance more toward praise with younger players whose self-esteem can be easily damaged.
- When communicating after a mistake, focus on the correction, not the mistake.
- Work on improving personal control of emotions.
- Learn to be a good listener.
- Learn to be a good questioner. Encourage players to self-reference, to assess themselves rather than always getting the coach's view. Ask, "How do you think you are doing?"
- Be aware of cultural differences and make allowances.

## THE KEY QUESTIONS A PLAYER NEEDS TO HAVE ANSWERED

- Why do you want me here?
- What is our team's purpose?
- What do you see as my special contribution?
- How will you make me a better player?
- How do you need me to prepare?
- What is my job on the field?
- What mentality do you want?
- What is the team game plan?
- What happens if I make a mistake?
- How will I be accountable for my performance?
- Can I trust you?
- Where do I go if I need help?

- Use players' names and know something of their families so you can express concern for them as people, not just players.
- Be prepared. Follow Stephen Covey's advice in knowing what outcome you want: "Begin with the end in mind" (1989, 97).
- Criticize only the performance, not the person.
- Avoid communicating when out of emotional control. Learn to wait for perspective and objectivity.
- Make maximum use of informal opportunities to communicate. A quiet word on the training ground often works better than a formal meeting.
- Use humor; fun is a great stress reliever.
- Always end communications by clarifying what you have agreed on: "So let's agree this is what we have decided to do."

It is unlikely that this helps a coach understand everything about their player's state of mind. However, the communication process does give player and coach a much better chance to close the gap and understand each other better. The more accurate the perception, the stronger the relationships are likely to be, and the better the chances of improved performance.

## Setting the Tone

Coaches should prepare for all meetings, but of special importance is the first meeting of a new coach and team when the coach must establish ground rules, attitude, and spirit. As the first significant team meeting, it will set the tone for both communication and relationships. The following is my advice to the head coach for the arrival-day meeting (45 minutes maximum):

- Offer a friendly welcome but move straight into an authoritative, businesslike manner reflecting your confidence and expertise.
- Insist from the start that the team concentrate, listen, and show respect for whoever is speaking (permit no mobile telephones).
- If possible, arrange a comfortable room with no distractions where players can all sit in a circle. This facilitates eye contact and indicates equal responsibility.
- Get any initial or potential problems out into the open to begin with, so players can listen with a clear mind. For example, ask, "Any problems with the rooms? Any problems with the food? Any health problems? Any other issues? OK, now we can begin."

*(continued)*

- Introduce your staff and indicate that each will speak for a few minutes after you have finished.
- Whenever possible, use players' names. Tell them what you and the staff wish to be called.
- Identify clearly the team's task and define what you will consider success.
- Remind the staff and players that they can only succeed through each other, that everybody is important.
- Share your vision of the way things should go. Offer a simple, clear, positive message that everyone can commit to.
- Remind players why they were selected and that they have a responsibility to live up to that honor. Indicate the standards, on and off the field, that are integral to any team.
- Review the obstacles that might prevent success.
- Talk the players through the preparation program (a visual aid and handouts of the schedule for the players will help). Gain their acceptance for the direction you intend to take them to ensure success.
- Ask if players have any questions so far. Listen carefully to any questions or comments.
- Talk openly and honestly about the things that directly or indirectly can affect team progress.
- Always use the word "we" to emphasize the shared nature of the exercise.
- Remind everyone of past success and the role that the experienced players in the group can play in helping the new players.
- End this first phase by reminding players of your vision of the way things should go.
- Introduce each member of the staff in turn and let them explain their roles in no more than two minutes each.
- Show a motivational film or find an inspirational message.

Conclude by linking the best practice of the film or message to your high expectations for this team.

# Summary

The profile of the modern coach inevitably will follow that of the modern player. One dramatic change in the modern player is an increasing demand for more and better communication that helps address personal performance and feelings about being a soccer player. Coaches can no longer handle players but must, as part of their player development program, build good relationships with each player. Players now seek coaches with good emotional intelligence and sensitive communication skills.

In order to deal with the fast-moving emotional roller coaster called a soccer season, coaches need to establish a communication network that players and coaches both understand and buy into. Both players and coaches might need help in both verbal and non-verbal communication as well as the use of modern technology. For coaches of young players, the use of e-mail and texting is a must.

Team meetings still offer coaches with good communication skills an effective and efficient way to get everybody on the same page while delivering a motivational boost. I visit many clubs with performance problems, and my first recommendation is increased and better communication networks. It is amazing how often this alone begins the process of improvement: "Increase communication; decrease anxiety."

# CHAPTER 10

# Role Definition: Team Tasks and Responsibilities

If you don't know what you are doing,
I can't put you in the game.

**Bill Belichick, head coach, New England Patriots**

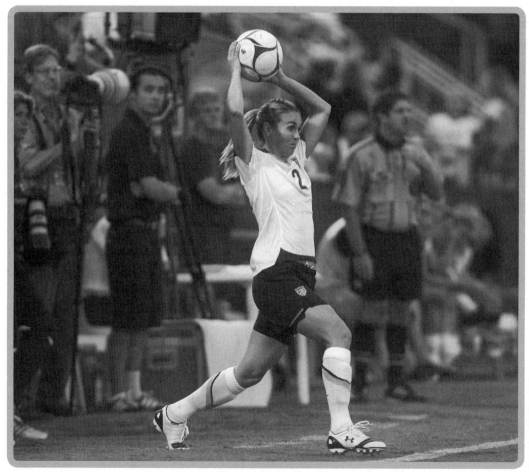

**A**ll players face performance anxiety, but one of the things that reassures them most in dealing with it is a belief that they know their job and can do it on the field. To help players establish mental clarity and confidence before a game, I urge them to focus, not on the bigger picture or the result, but instead on reachable goals. I ask the players to concentrate hard on the three things that they can do in their position for the team; plus I remind them to be a good team member and support their teammates. Thus it is vital that coaches see role definition as a key part of player development. While I understand the argument for role flexibility with younger players, having a regular position and role definition becomes more important as players get older and the level of play improves.

Coaches who swap players positionally in order to solve tactical or selection issues forget that they are giving the players problems that could result in a loss of confidence. This happens from time to time with one of England's best centerbacks when asked to cover the fullback position "in order to help the team out." Every time he is moved from a position he loves, knows, and is confident about to a position that leaves him feeling exposed and unsure, he feels anger, disappointment, and anxiety. Coaches who select the best players and then try to fit them into their positional system may find that putting round pegs in square holes may lead to a loss of confidence and a very unsure performance.

The responsibility of the coach is to ensure mental clarity and emotional balance by preparing players for their roles in empathic, interesting, and challenging ways. Good coaches reduce complexity for players, a process known as the reduction of uncertainty.

Although all positions share certain fundamental requirements, coaches must be able to teach special skills and responsibilities for various positions. If the player knows that the coach has a real understanding of her position, she will be far more willing to accept criticism of her performance. This helps maintain a good coach–player relationship. Michelle Akers, a leading player on the U.S. women's world championship team, demands such analysis and attention to detail from her coaches:

> Coaches must extend women players as much as the guys. It's no good telling a girl "well done," when she's lost control and trapped the ball a few yards out in front of her. I divide my goals into the following categories—fitness, technique, mental, position-specific, and diet.

Another advantage of having job descriptions is that coaches can more easily recognize mismatches between role demands and player abilities. Darren Edmondson at Carlisle was a failing midfield player, a clear mismatch, until it was recognized that his abilities matched those of a fullback. He became a much more productive player at his new position. Similarly, Sir Geoff Hurst, scorer of a hat trick in the 1966 World Cup final, was converted from a failing midfield player into a world-class striker. In this age of technological advancement, the use of improved match analysis and film evidence has made it far easier for coaches and players to match job descriptions with actual performance. This then allows for higher quality feedback and subsequent specific training.

# Field Position and Player Profile

To help players with their positional role, coaches themselves have to build a general role profile for each position. Clearly each position brings its own particular emphasis on the characteristics required for success. Table 10.1 selects one position—central midfield (primarily acting as sweeper in front of a back line of four defenders)—and illustrates one way of building a complete profile of characteristics required. This process must test positional responsibilities in these situations:

● In attack
● In defense
● In transition
● At set pieces
● In a variety of "what if" game scenarios

In building this profile coaches are also helping pinpoint their future recruiting needs.

| TABLE 10.1—Positional Profile: Central Midfield Player | |
|---|---|
| **Performance areas** | **Key qualities** |
| Physical | Strong physical presence, intimidating, durable (doesn't become injured easily), good stamina, quick over short distances, good jumping ability to win headers, outstanding work ethic |
| Technical | Has excellent quick control (always playing in traffic), can pass short with high certainty and long with accuracy, can join the attack, has good long shot, understands that simplicity is excellence for this role |
| Tactical | Team player, understands gameplan, excellent in transition play, team organizer, recognizes dangerous situations, good communicator, sees whole field, covers for others |
| Mental | Good learner, quick thinker, decisive, tough-minded, highly disciplined, resilient (recovers from mistakes), accepts responsibility, outstanding concentration, intelligent reader of game situations |
| Emotional | Calm, composed presence at heart of the team, has excellent self-control and is good at leading teammates, never intimidated or provoked, deals with stress well, is trustworthy, a potential captain |
| Lifestyle | Dedicated athlete with lifestyle to match, will not abuse body, conscientious about game preparation, does not seek glory or headlines |

## Technology, Coach Round, and Stewart Downing

I was impressed at Middlesbrough by the way coach Steve Round helped his young, left wide midfield player, Stewart Downing, appreciate the demands of his position and role on the field. Coach Round asked Prozone Ltd for the average game statistics of the top five percent of players in the Premier League in Stewart's position. He then used these statistics to both educate and motivate Stewart by showing him where he compared well and where he could improve.

| Left wide midfield player | Premier League average (top 5%) | Stewart's ranking |
|---|---|---|
| Distance covered | 13 kilometers | Top 2 |
| High-speed runs | 1,500 meters | Top 2 |
| Number of sprints | 60 | Top 2 |
| Passes received | 65+ | Top 3 |
| Passes retained | 80+ percent | Top 5 |
| Crosses | 6-10 | Top 1 |
| Strikes | 4 per game | Top 3 |
| Goals | 5 per season | Top 5 |
| Tackles won | 2 | – |
| Headers won | 2 | – |

Note: Stewart's statistics were in the top 5 percent for his position in most respects, but clearly, though an excellent player, he needed to work on tackling and headers won. Stewart recognized this and has worked very hard to improve his defensive duties.

# Building a Job Description

It is important that coaches are clear on their expectations and standards for each player in each position before they engage with their players. Having identified the performance profile for each position, coaches can now be more specific about their job description for each position. Although the coach will have a clear idea of what he wants from each position in relation to the tactical system, building a job description does offer a chance to share ownership by including players in the process. Table 10.2 (page 158) reflects the views of the centerbacks and fullbacks at Middlesbrough when asked to profile their specific job descriptions.

| TABLE 10.2—Fullbacks' and Centerbacks' Views of Their Job Descriptions | |
|---|---|
| **Fullback job description** | **Centerback job description** |
| **1.** Attitude<br>• Be aggressive; win 90 percent of all challenges.<br>• Win our 1v1 battle.<br>• Be mentally disciplined; concentrate 90+ minutes.<br>• Be very fit; we defend and attack. | **1.** Attitude<br>• Be aggressive; win 90 percent of all our challenges.<br>• Be determined; defend and win your 1v1.<br>• Stay calm and composed; we are always in control. |
| **2.** Attacking<br>• Be positive; always take the ball.<br>• Support, provide and build a partnership with the wide man.<br>• Overlap; create 2v1 and make crosses. | **2.** Attacking<br>• Be reliable in possession; minimum 70 percent pass completion rate<br>• Maintain continuity; provide for those who can score.<br>• Switch play; stretch through diagonal passes. |
| **3.** Defending<br>• Position; read the game.<br>• Stay tight on my side and cover on opposite side.<br>• Stop the crosses.<br>• Communicate; see along the line. | **3.** Defending<br>• Read the game, position early and anticipate.<br>• Have passion to defend well; be first to the ball.<br>• Concentrate; be a 90+ minutes team player<br>• Know the opposition; take away their threat.<br>• Stay fit, strong, and agile; we sacrifice to meet the challenge. |
|  | **4.** Leadership<br>• Be disciplined; stay out of the red (stay composed).<br>• Organize and communicate.<br>• Commit: we demand from ourselves and others |
| *Defend. Support. Provide.*<br>Play hard. Play soccer. Play together. | The team *trusts* us to be *reliable.*<br>Play hard. Play soccer. Play together. |

Of course the exercise can continue on into more specific detail according to the needs of the players. These exercises produce the following conditions:

● A shared agreement on job role and responsibilities

● A common language of communication: coach–player, player–player

● A framework for more specific performance analysis and feedback

● A vehicle for holding the player more accountable

● A challenge for the coach's ability to teach soccer

At the very least, the interaction between player and coach helps democratize their relationship, an important element for the modern player. When the player and coach share an understanding of the player's role, several benefits will become evident:

- Communication increases, and anxiety decreases.
- The player feels that his experience and knowledge are valued.
- The player understands his strengths and weaknesses.
- The player self-references and takes responsibility for his performance.
- The danger of asking the player to do things beyond his capability is reduced.
- The player is accountable in a more objective manner, reducing the chance of unfair criticism from the coach.
- Mutual respect increases.

Thus the player and coach both have the critical information they need to do their jobs under the pressure and demands of the game. Just as important, shared ownership stimulates the player's emotional attachment to the team. A new player, or a dissatisfied player, who buys into the idea of shared ownership will naturally become integrated with the ambitions and structure of the team. Bill Walsh summarized the process:

> By establishing his role on the team and taking pride in the fact he is contributing in a tangible way, a rookie can achieve a sense of control in his professional life. Not only is he able to earn his "keep," he is also able to acquire the acceptance of his teammates. (1998)

## Strikers and Goalkeepers

One of my special roles at the clubs I work with is giving support to the strikers and goalkeepers. These players are special because they more often than not define the game and so carry the burden of extra responsibility. They also carry the high expectations of their families, coaches, teammates, fans, and the media, and in each game either succeed or fail to meet these expectations, with not much in between. Every coach in the world is looking to recruit the most talented of these players.

For a sport psychologist helping coaches deal with performance issues, strikers and goalkeepers offer a range of interesting psychological issues:

- They are special to the coach.
- They define the game, win or lose.
- They are always under pressure.
- They emotionally crave success.

● Their mistakes are easily observed.

● They are an easy target for criticism.

● Their life is highs and lows.

● They suffer constantly changing self-esteem.

One of the starting points for dealing with these issues—and note how many have clear psychological implications—is a clear job description agreed upon between goalkeepers or strikers and their coaches. At the start of the season, I meet with the player and his coach, and we share the process of defining what exact performance we expect, and therefore what preparation the player should concentrate on. For example, in building a job description for a striker, I encourage the coach and player to work from the end backward:

● The most important function of the striker is to score goals.

● The next most important function is to create goals.

● To do this, the striker must get into the penalty box as often as possible (90 percent of goals are scored here).

● To help build up the play that allows them to get into the box and receive balls, the striker must hold up passes played forward, link play, and allow his team to move up the field with good possession.

● When the ball is lost, the striker becomes the front line of a team defense, applying pressure to win the ball back.

● All of that takes a tough, competitive attitude: hard work, courage, aggressiveness, power, speed, sharpness, and resilience.

Table 10.3 shows the resultant job description for a striker.

| **TABLE 10.3—Job Description for a Striker** | |
| --- | --- |
| **1.** Attitude | • Pressure the ball.<br>• Take the ball.<br>• Take the hits.<br>• Take the shot. |
| **2.** Hold the ball up | • Allow team to move up.<br>• Keep possession. |
| **3.** Get into the box | • Employ the skill.<br>• Exploit movement.<br>• Create freedom. |
| **4.** Create a goal | • Create time and space for teammates. |
| **5.** Score a goal | |
| If I miss, I only think: *I will get the next one.* | |

| TABLE 10.4—Positional Profile: Goalkeeper | |
|---|---|
| **Performance areas** | **Key qualities** |
| Physical | **1.** Strength<br>**2.** Athleticism (agility)<br>**3.** Presence (stature)<br>**4.** Fitness (endurance)<br>**5.** Diet (well-being) |
| Technical | **1.** Handling<br>**2.** Distribution (feet and hands)<br>**3.** Dealing with crosses<br>**4.** Starting position and general positioning<br>**5.** Quick feet (dealing with back passes) |
| Tactical | **1.** Knowing and reading the game<br>**2.** Decision-making (speed of thought)<br>**3.** Communication (staying alert)<br>**4.** Control of teammates (penalty area)<br>**5.** Distribution (setting the tempo) |
| Mental | **1.** Positive attitude<br>**2.** Confidence (good self-image)<br>**3.** Toughness (determination)<br>**4.** Focus (concentration—94 minutes)<br>**5.** Bravery (enjoy the challenge) |
| Emotional | **1.** Control (positive self-talk)<br>**2.** Clear mind (relaxed and composed)<br>**3.** Handling mistakes (recovery skills)<br>**4.** Enduring self-belief<br>**5.** Peace of mind (home, family, work, and self) |
| Lifestyle | **1.** Being professional in all things<br>**2.** Stable home life<br>**3.** Disciplined care of the body<br>**4.** Avoiding celebrity temptations<br>**5.** Switching on and switching off (leaving the game on the field) |

Table 10.4, a profile of a goalkeeper's job, reflects the thoughts of Mark Schwarzer, the Australian international, and his goalkeeping colleagues when at Middlesbrough.

Once such job descriptions are agreed upon, they act as very clear and objective targets for performance and ensure relevant feedback and accountability. Again the process of shared ownership ensures player cooperation and improves coach–player relationships.

Using the job description exercise as a starting point, I asked Paul Barron, a top goalkeeping coach, and Steve Round, one of the best striker coaches I have worked with, to explain their player–coach relationship. Paul Barron builds his relationship with his goalkeepers with the following:

1. Offering constant unwavering support
2. Engaging in everyday communication
3. Being honest about good news and bad news
4. Showing concern for them as human beings
5. Being strong for them in the bad times

Steve Round describes the following priorities for creating good relationships with his strikers:

1. Being positive and available
2. Forgiving mistakes and moving on quickly
3. Understanding ego and managing moods
4. Showing respect and being a good listener
5. Celebrating and reinforcing success

## I'll Get the Next One

When Newcastle played away at Derby, their famous striker, Alan Shearer, was presented in the first minute with a clear one-on-one with the Derby goalkeeper. Much to the surprise of everybody and the amusement of the Derby crowd, Alan made a complete mess of the opportunity. Eighty-six minutes later with the game 0-0, Alan received a second opportunity from a wide free kick. This time he chested the ball down and volleyed a spectacular goal from 20 meters—the winning goal!

When asked what he was thinking after his early mistake Alan answered: "Same as always – I'll get the next one."

Alan's mental toughness as a striker, ready to deal with his mistakes and stay focused and committed (a key part of his job description), enabled him to be ready to deal with the next opportunity and win the game for his team.

# Ten Steps to Developing a Player's Ability to Perform a Role

By now, coaches have established a performance profile for each position within their tactical framework. With this clearly in mind, and checked against every possible phase of the game (attacking, defending, set plays, and so on), the coach can now engage each player in understanding her specific role. Together they can build a job description that helps the player understand what is expected of her and by what performance measures she will be held accountable. Coaches can then help players by establishing the right learning environment:

*1. Specific learning and development*   Decide what the player must learn in order to do her job superbly, assessing the demands for her specific position.

*2. Assess the player*   How does the player's present level of physical, technical, tactical, mental, and emotional capacity fit the requirements of the job? Identify the weaknesses that require special attention.

*3. Design relevant practice*   Apart from the general work every player needs, what does this player especially need to practice for this particular job?

*4. Bias practice for success*   Lead the player forward in a series of small, manageable steps that create an atmosphere of success and show the player that training pays off.

*5. Give criticism with care*   The player will need ongoing evaluation (coaching is the reduction of errors), but it must be positive and productive, encouraging the player to deal with mistakes and criticism as a necessary part of the learning process.

*6. Treat setbacks as part of the journey*   If it were easy, everybody would play soccer well. But it isn't, so the player must be prepared for setbacks. The coach must retain emotional control and focus on the learning process and error reduction. The clever coach will use such errors as a guide to preparing for future practices, thereby ensuring relevance.

*7. Share ownership with the player*   If the player feels involved from the start of the process, it is more likely that she will find the commitment to see it through to the end. The coach must encourage the player to share her views. Both must be willing to deal with bad news as well as good.

*8. Use "best practice" models*   Players often learn faster and more easily if they have a role model to emulate. Young players who watch a star player on film playing just the way the coach wants them to play are soon convinced. Similarly, a coach may take a player to a game so that both of them can concentrate on and learn from the play of a role model. For example, they might watch the player's work rate and contribution without the ball.

*9. Evaluate progress*   Players must see that they are improving if they are to stay motivated, so coaches should seek any measures available to do this. These might include the following:

- Objective statistics—for example, the number of clean sheets for a goalkeeper

- Subjective reports—a compilation of the player's view, the coach's view, and the views of independent experts
- Film clips—evidence that the player can see for herself
- External approval—promotion to a higher team, selection for the national team, or media recognition

*10. Reward progress*   Coaches must look for players doing things right and reward any sign of improvement. The only way to create good habits is by constant repetition. To provide repetition without boredom, the coach must vary practices. The player needs the constant encouragement of both the coach and her social support group, avoiding any cynics and moaners among family and friends.

## The Player's Role Within a Team

In a team game like soccer, players must do more than simply understand and perform their individual roles; they must do so within a cohesive pattern of 11 players either attacking or defending at any particular stage of the game. For advanced tactical systems, for example, the total soccer of former Holland teams, players may be asked to interchange positions. The successful team player must take four steps in developing his particular role:

1. Understand and perform his role as a primary contribution to the team.
2. Form a unit with the players who play nearby and perform in coordination with them. This is sometimes known as teams within teams.
3. Understand the tactical shape of the whole team and how his particular role contributes to team success.
4. Be willing to accept any amendments to the role that the coaches determine necessary to win a particular game.

As these steps unfold, the coach might find the player resistant to change. The coach will have to employ more skills to reorient the player from personal goals to team goals. Occasionally I like to quote Rudyard Kipling:

> Now this is the law of the jungle
> As old and as true as the sky
> And the wolf that keeps it may prosper
> And the wolf that shall break it must die
> As the creeper that circles the tree trunk
> The law runneth forward and back
> The strength of the pack is the wolf
> **And the strength of the wolf is the pack** [emphasis added]. (Kipling, "The Law of the Jungle," stanza 1)

Symbols like this are useful in encouraging togetherness and reinforcing the concept that the team is the hero. Blending players' roles and responsibilities into a cohesive team is not easy. The case study "Soldier or Artist?" tries to illustrate the varied nature of players and what each can offer if the coach can identify an appropriate role. Soldier-artists or artist-soldiers are relatively easy to fit within the team concept, but pure soldiers or pure artists can give the coach headaches. If the coach–player relationship is sound, however, a role might be shaped that the player can accept and, just as important, that the rest of the team can see as beneficial to their chances of success.

Steve McClaren, head coach of FC Twente in Holland, always tries to include an artist at number 10 in his teams. At his former club, Middlesbrough, Steve built the team around Juninho, and now at FC Twente, he's

## Soldier or Artist?

Dave Sexton, one of England's most distinguished former coaches, once remarked that a soccer team includes soldiers and artists. When I had the opportunity to work alongside Coach Sexton, I questioned him further. He felt that all players could be identified somewhere along a continuum:

Soldier          Soldier-artist          Artist-soldier          Artist

- The soldier is combative in nature, physically powerful, a natural defender or perhaps an abrasive attacker.
- The soldier-artist is similar to the soldier but with a touch of vision and skill that occasionally produces unexpected finesse.
- The artist-soldier is predominantly a player of vision and skill but could surprise everybody with the ability to compete strongly for the ball.
- The artist is a player of the highest skill levels, capable of making brilliant, insightful decisions on the pitch and forever seeking to make things happen, but often negligent and weak on defensive duties.

Coach Sexton felt it was important for each player to know his natural style and what he could contribute. It was also important, Sexton believed, for the coach to place players in roles within a team shape that allowed them to express their style and talents.

Pure soldiers are easy to place in a role but will have limited ability to make a mark at the highest levels. Pure artists are prized but less easy to place in an efficient and effective role in competitive soccer played at the highest level. For total soccer and the complete team, any coach would love a combination of soldier-artists and artist-soldiers, all of whom would find roles to suit them in a physically competitive team capable of moments of real skill and flair.

built the team around Kenny Perez, both outstanding artists. This is not an easy coaching situation and can only happen if

- the coach truly believes in what the artist brings to the team;
- the rest of the team is balanced to support the artist's strengths and cover for his weaknesses;
- what the artist brings to the team is seen as important, and he feels loved; and
- the coach has the courage to live with mistakes (being creative is not easy) and wait for the defining moments that artists can create that influence the success of the team.

# Summary

One of the foundations of a player's competitive toughness and confidence is a clear understanding of his job on the field. When this job description is built with the guidance of the coach, the coach–player relationship becomes much stronger.

This chapter emphasizes that one of the most important exercises coaches can do with his players is to build and agree on a job description that covers player responsibility in all phases of play. Examples included cover various field positions, but strikers and goalkeepers are highlighted as needing special support in understanding and doing their job on the field. These two positions carry great responsibility, often defining the game, and so their job descriptions and resultant coach–player understanding becomes a very important antidote to the pressure.

The chapter concludes by offering coaches 10 key steps to developing a player's ability to perform his role on the field. Creating role definition and a joint job description remains a key step in both tactical and mental progress and the development of a sound coach–player relationship.

# CHAPTER 11

# Cohesion: Building a Coordinated Team

All of the efforts to build cohesive team relationships and a strong team experience are for moments when the challenges and demands are at their absolute greatest and when nothing short of our best is demanded. And in that moment, we must understand that we are in it together, that we are one great big family together, and that we are the greatest team in the world!

**Sue Humphrey, U.S. women's track and field coach, in Taylor and Wilson (2005)**

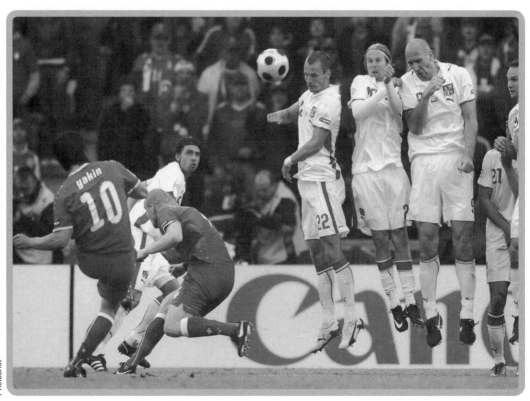

When Coach Pat Riley moved from the championship-winning Los Angeles Lakers to the New York Knicks, he found a team battling against itself. Team cohesion had broken down, and the players operated either alone or in small groups. When the players arrived for their first meeting with Coach Riley, he had organized the room into a number of groups of chairs representing the players' friendship groups. Each player was directed to a specific chair, and then the coach asked the players to look around the room. He told them that a team divided cannot win and then left them for fifteen minutes to consider their options. When Coach Riley returned, the players had re-formed the room into a semicircle of chairs with one left for the coach. In just one meeting, the coach had moved the players from a "me" culture to a "we" culture and begun the process of building team cohesion and winning (Riley 1993).

The science and art of building teams and team cohesion are the key challenge of soccer. To release the power of their individual players, the coach has to drive home the following messages:

- We achieve more when we agree to work together.
- We achieve more when we encourage each other.
- We achieve more when we accept responsibility for our role.

When players accept this and engage in a team process, they release their talent and power in a way they could not individually. Cohesive teams seem to generate greater power and presence on the field and certainly deal with adversity better. Creating such teams, however, is not easy, as Pat Riley outlines:

> Teamwork isn't simple. In fact, it can be a frustrating, elusive commodity. That's why there are so many bad teams out there, stuck in neutral or going downhill. Teamwork doesn't appear magically, just because someone mouths the words. It doesn't thrive just because of the presence of talent or ambition. It doesn't flourish simply because a team has tasted success. (16)

Team building and teamwork occur only as the result of strategic development by an experienced coach and the voluntary commitment of players who are engaged and drawn in by the process. Both are essential to team success. Great teams are characterised by both the quality of leadership and the ability and commitment of the players.

## The Challenge for the Coach

The coach is instrumental to team cohesion because he is the central point of all communication and has the power and authority to make changes. To maintain such cohesion under the pressure of a soccer season, the coach must display a consistent approach to players and their contribution to the team. The coach's philosophy and style must emphasize a culture of "we," not "me," and togetherness. Soccer is not a one-on-one sport, but an eleven-on-eleven sport. Teams succeed when coaches maximize players' potential by getting them to coordinate their individual talents into a cohesive team operation.

In 2004, the U.S. Olympic basketball team had the best individual players but lacked cohesion and the balance of outside shooters. When their opponents saw this, they blocked up the middle and allowed the outside shot, and the United States, with the most talent, lost their way.

In Lavin's (2005) analysis of how coach Bill Belichick built success with the New England Patriots, he reinforces the philosophy of team first. Even after winning the Super Bowl, Belichick stressed that the trophy was for the team and not for outstanding individual performers.

Like Belichick, a coach must have leadership qualities and must be an inspirational role model who can win the respect of players, create a future vision that excites the team, and create an environment in which players willingly sacrifice and play for each other. Creating a team vision—a picture of what's possible, a destination that excites players, and a reason why everybody should work hard and persevere—is fundamental to team cohesion. The great team builders

- create a vision that can bind the team together;
- get the team to buy into it;
- repeat the vision regularly during the season, but often in different forms; and
- produce the agreed vision whenever cohesion is threatened.

Table 11.1 (page 170) offers guidelines to help coaches with the challenge of building team cohesion.

## The Challenge for the Player

Personal agendas, of course, are important for players, and it is the clever coach who works hard to give players the rewards, identity, care, and attention they are seeking. This clears the way for the coach to persuade the players to commit to a team philosophy. This is never more difficult than when dealing with the star player. A combination of strong coaching plus pressure from teammates can be the only factors that prevent a personality player from threatening team cohesion. The player who cannot make the move from "me" to "we" suffers what Pat Riley aptly calls the "disease of me" (1993). When this disease spreads through the team, several conditions can occur:

- Collapse of team commitment
- Team sabotage (loss of emotional balance)

| **TABLE 11.1—Guidelines for Building Team Cohesion** |
|---|
| Establish a team credo, a description that is binding. |
| Sell the dream and share ownership with the players. |
| Establish honesty and trust between players and coaches. |
| Show composure on all issues and maintain emotional balance. |
| Make playing for your team special; create image and identity. |
| Maximize the value of anything positive that happens. |
| Minimize the impact of anything negative. |
| Increase communication and decrease anxiety. |
| Build a player core by continuity of selection and loyalty. |
| Challenge all players to be the best they can be. |
| Seek leadership from within the team. |
| Build togetherness through the hard work of preparation. |
| Be proactive in dealing with problems. |
| Use bonding exercises to create team chemistry. |
| Learn from every experience; embrace victory or defeat. |
| Constantly feed the players images of success. |
| Balance work, rest, and recovery. |
| Demonstrate this positive approach with all the staff involved with the team. |
| Control the environment, allowing in only what helps. |

- The team divided
- The team doing just enough to get by
- Players who create 20 percent of the results believing they deserve 80 percent of the rewards

When Michael Jordan first joined the Chicago Bulls basketball team, Coach Phil Jackson recognized his unique talent but also saw the effect it was having on the rest of the team. Michael was so good and wanted the ball so much that the other players suffered a decline in motivation and perceived status. The team began to lose cohesion and games.

The problem was solved by a remark from Coach Jackson's mentor, veteran coach Tex Winter, who described Jordan as good but not great. Michael demanded to know why, and Coach Winter explained that good players on teams become great only when they make the players around them better. Once Michael absorbed this, he adapted his game to involve his teammates more. The players came together behind his leadership, and a championship team was born. So the challenge for the team player is to give up some aspects of a personal agenda—recognition, comfort, or rewards—to meet the needs of a team agenda and the potential return of even greater success. The successful coach will identify and take care of each player's personal agenda in order to persuade him to commit to the team philosophy.

The highly respected Dutch soccer coach and team builder Rinus Michels (1996) describes team building as a structured process in which the coach sets parameters and encourages player involvement but emphasizes that the quality and maturity of the players finally determines the destiny of the team. This is the reason I believe cohesive teams contain influential senior players, a core group who have matured with experience and whose presence can give the team character and stability. American football coach Chuck Noll confirms this:

> On every team there is a core group that sets the tone for everybody else. If the tone is positive, you have half the battle won. If negative, you are beaten before you ever walk on the field. (Walsh 1998)

## Team Stability—Mental and Emotional Issues

Having now experienced fourteen seasons with five professional teams in the most competitive soccer league in the world, I have witnessed all the stages of team building and the situations and incidents that conspire to destroy the process. The key to my work is establishing a mature mental and emotional stability in the team that allows for consistent performance with the positive support of the players. Each week, the events of soccer—an unexpected loss, a key injury, the departure of a player, disagreements on selection, conflict between players, and so on—threaten the stability of the team and undermine its will to commit to the cause. Daniel Goleman, a leading expert on emotional intelligence—the capacity for recognizing our own feelings and those of others—reinforces this:

> Collective emotional intelligence is what sets top performing teams apart from average teams. Group emotional intelligence determines a team's ability to manage its emotions in a way that cultivates trust, group identity, and group efficiency and so maximizes cooperation, collaboration, and effectiveness. (2002, 177)

Goleman suggested that harmony was most negatively affected by players who were either deadweights or dominators; players who couldn't cope with the give and take of a team plus the insidious effect of the emotions of fear, anger, rivalry, and resentment. Generally, in teams that lack cohesion, everybody worries about people not doing their jobs. Thus, the challenge of becoming a successful team member is far more likely to be emotional than it is physical. The soccer of tomorrow will require players to have the basic elements of a mature well-developed emotional intelligence so that they can play effectively in a team situation. To succeed in the toughest leagues and tournaments, teams will need to boost their collective emotional intelligence and achieve a high degree of stability.

Much of my work in preparing England teams for international play has been directed at establishing the emotional intelligence and stability that allows physical skills to flourish in unfamiliar and difficult environments. Limited preparation time makes this difficult. Figure 11.1 shows this role in supporting and linking the triangle of relationships. Because I know everybody's viewpoint, when stability is threatened, I can be proactive by suggesting changes that defuse the situation. This echoes the belief of Ian McGeechan, coach of the British Lions rugby team on their tour of South Africa, who felt that if he got the psychology right, everything else would fall into place.

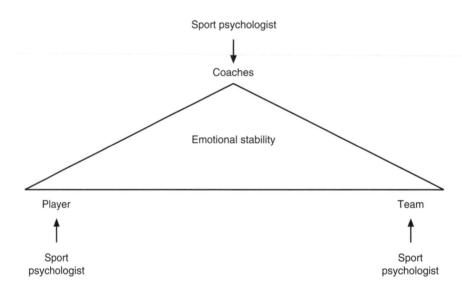

**FIGURE 11.1**   Sport psychologist's role in creating team stability.

## Building Team Cohesion

Maintaining the psychological stability of a team at a good performance level throughout a long season or a challenging tournament is the result of the team's cohesion. This is built on two main foundations: task cohesion and social cohesion.

## Task Cohesion

Task cohesion refers to the extent to which a team is able to play in an efficient, effective, and coordinated manner. Coaches and players agree on the way the team intends to play. All players on the team should be comfortable with their

- own positional role and responsibilities;
- job as part of a team unit; for example, as part of the front two strikers;
- job as part of the overall team game plan; and
- job in special situations, such as set plays or "what if" scenarios.

This demands the following from the coach:

1. Philosophy: a clear philosophy on how he wants the game to be played.
2. Strategy: the ability to break the overall game plan down into both phases of play and how team units operate, and individual play giving each player accurate job descriptions.
3. Teaching: the ability to communicate and teach these messages every day.

The great teaching skill of coaching is being able to break the full game into parts more easily taught, repeat them in practice until the quality improves, and then re-integrate them in to the game successfully. The great coaches are often the great teachers, and Steve Jamison regards the late football coach Bill Walsh as one of the best.

> Bill Walsh was an educator—a teacher. He accumulated great knowledge because he was a grade A student of leadership, paying close attention along the way to some of football's most outstanding and forward-thinking coaches. Bill absorbed their good ideas, learned from their bad ones, applied his even more advanced concepts, and then reveled in the process of teaching what he knew to his teams. He loved it. (Walsh 2009, xxvii)

Players derive much of their confidence on game day from a feeling of being fully prepared and knowing exactly what the coach expects of them. Tom Landry, the former American football coach, understood this perfectly. As he famously stated, "I don't believe in team motivation. I believe in getting a team prepared so it knows it will have the necessary confidence when it steps on the field and be prepared to play a good game."

Coaches will quickly identify lack of task cohesion when they see problems in team shape, coordination, communication, motivation, and concentration. Table 11.2 (page 174) allows each coach to assess the team's present level of task cohesion. The more assessments a coach can gather, the more likely he is to have a valid picture. Clearly, an action plan for change is needed in areas of little or no understanding.

## TABLE 11.2—Assessing Your Team's Level of Task Cohesion

Assess, as a coaching staff, how well your team understands how to deal with these game situations.

| Game situation | Full understanding | Some understanding | No understanding |
|---|---|---|---|
| • Each player knows his individual job. | | | |
| • Each player understands his unit job (e.g., back four, midfield, and so on). | | | |
| • Each player understands the team game plan. | | | |
| • Each player knows and is enthusiastic about the team targets. | | | |
| • Each player is prepared at | | | |
|    – our kickoffs, | | | |
|    – their kickoffs, | | | |
|    – our goal kicks, | | | |
|    – their goal kicks, | | | |
|    – our corners, | | | |
|    – their corners, | | | |
|    – our free kicks, | | | |
|    – their free kicks, | | | |
|    – our throw-ins | | | |
|    – their throw-ins | | | |
| • Each player understands how to play after we score. | | | |
| • Each player understands how to play after they score. | | | |
| • Each player knows his job when we are chasing the game. | | | |
| • Each player knows his job when we are defending a lead. | | | |
| • Each player understands how to play when we or they are down to 10 players. | | | |
| • Each player knows how to play when on a yellow card. | | | |

From B. Beswick, 2010, *Focused for Soccer, Second Edition* (Champaign, IL: Human Kinetics).

## Social Cohesion

Coaches must always remember they are dealing with human beings as well as human actions, and their strategy for team cohesion must include a personal factor. The art of coaching includes building relationships with players so they want to play for you, and encouraging player-player relationships so they want to play for each other. Task cohesion will provide the route to effective soccer productivity, but it is social cohesion that can deliver the extra energy and engagement.

If coaches are to engage modern young players and compete with all the lifestyle and choice issues their generation possesses, then they must see relationship coaching and social cohesion as key skills. Table 11.3 (page 176) allows the coach to assess the team's level of social cohesion. Depending on the particular situation, coaches may use support staff, parents, and players to offer a wider range of assessments. Statements answered as "some truth" or "false" offer coaches early warning of team issues and the chance to effect change.

In teams with social cohesion, the players can relate and communicate with each other, are capable of solving problems, and can remain unified in identity and purpose. Lack of social cohesion can lead to problems of players who will not play together, will not play for each other, and will not bond together.

Building cohesion is not easy because successful performance in highly competitive situations is a complex and fragile process requiring careful planning and patience. Sometimes teams that are not cohesive will win because of their talent, but this will not happen consistently. On the other hand, teams with less talent can often win games by maximizing the cohesive purpose and synergy of the team.

Successful performance requires a team to do many things right on a consistent and integrated basis. It is only through pursuing an active strategy of task and social cohesion that the coach can hope to achieve that. Similarly, players must examine their own qualities and ensure that they can be full and contributing members of such a process.

# The Relationship Between Task and Social Cohesion

The relationship, and relative importance, of task and social cohesion varies with the status and objectives of the team. Coaches need to clearly define what business they are in for their particular team. One of the key lessons coaches must learn is to lead and manage according to the context they are working in. The age, level, and gender characteristics of their team immediately define and limit both coaching philosophy and style.

| TABLE 11.3—Assessing Your Team's Level of Social Cohesion | | | |
|---|---|---|---|
| Assess, as a coaching staff, how well your team scores on the following situations. | | | |
| **Situation** | **True** | **Some truth** | **False** |
| • Players enjoy playing for our team. | | | |
| • Very few players leave our team willingly. | | | |
| • We have a high level of communication. | | | |
| • It's hard work but fun to be on our team. | | | |
| • Our team is never bored. | | | |
| • Players on our team grow as people. | | | |
| • Ethnic and cultural differences are not important on our team. | | | |
| • Players respect, appreciate, and encourage each other. | | | |
| • We have stars but no isolates. | | | |
| • We have a good record of developing player leadership. | | | |
| • Honesty and trust are key words for us. | | | |
| • We deal quickly with players who disrupt team harmony. | | | |
| • Setbacks and defeats do not undermine morale. | | | |
| • We surround our players with good, positive adults. | | | |
| • Parents are part of the solution, not the problem. | | | |
| • Togetherness is a key theme in all our meetings. | | | |
| • Coach–coach relationships are positive and respectful. | | | |

From B. Beswick, 2010, *Focused for Soccer, Second Edition* (Champaign, IL: Human Kinetics).

Such understanding may lead to a differing emphasis on task and social cohesion, as illustrated:

***Example 1: Recreational Soccer***   In a team of young people or a recreational group, social cohesion might assume more importance than task cohesion. "The main thing is to enjoy being together."

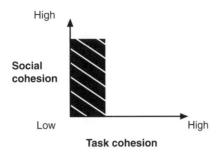

**Example 2: Professional Soccer**  In a professional team or a team whose stated objective is to win, then task cohesion assumes more importance than social cohesion. "I don't have to like you to play with you if you help me win."

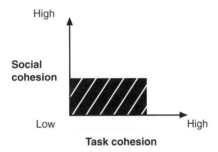

**Example 3: Soccer Excellence**  The best route to a winning state of mind and sustainable soccer excellence is through very high levels of task cohesion supported by a drive to establish and promote positive relationships. "We're a happy team that works hard on its game."

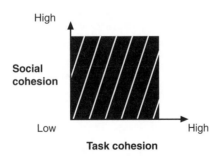

For the most part, coaches and players enter the challenge of soccer with a desire to achieve, and so the emphasis should be on task cohesion and performance. As significant performance results are achieved, social cohesion should be a natural by-product of players learning to trust, like, and respect each other.

# Team Cohesion in Women's Soccer

All coaches understand the power of a cohesive team of 11 players working hard and going in the same direction, but for coaches of womens' teams, the process of building such cohesion, while equally challenging, is different. Whereas the coaches of men will focus immediately on task cohesion and let relationships occur as a by-product, coaches of women must make relationship coaching and social cohesion the starting point for any team development. When a female player joins a team, one of her primary needs is social acceptance and affirmation of her role within the team. Kathleen DeBoer stresses the difference between the needs of men and women:

> The task orientation of males means they bond and form alliances through shared activity; the relationship orientation of females means they bond and form alliances through conversation. (2008, 25)

> DeBoer describes this process as "Male: struggle—performance—acceptance" and "Female: acceptance—struggle—performance" (34).

In general, women play for each other, stick up for each other, don't like being singled out—either positively or negatively—and expect their coaches to be emotionally intelligent. This social contract, a sense of belonging and togetherness, must be in place before coaches can focus on competitive challenge. Once that social cohesion is in place, coaches of women's teams will find that their players will work very hard to improve.

## Breaking the Social Contract

The U.S. women's soccer team lost 4-0 to Brazil in the 2007 World Cup competition when the social contract—and therefore team cohesion—broke down. The U.S. coach, thinking strategically rather than psychologically, replaced an established goalkeeper (who had not been scored on for nearly 300 minutes) with a back-up keeper who had had previous success against Brazil. The coach's one-dimensional thinking missed out a key question: "What impact will this have on the rest of the team?" Clearly, the team judged this unfair, togetherness was disturbed, team harmony disrupted, and the team unsettled enough to record a shocking defeat.

## THE CORE COVENANT

*Every team that wants to move forward to significance and greatness has to decide what truths and values it will be bound by—co-operation, love, hard work, total concentration—for the good of the team. This covenant is an agreement that*

- *binds players together,*
- *creates equal footing,*
- *helps players shoulder their responsibilities,*
- *prescribes terms for the help and support of others, and*
- *creates a foundation for teamwork.*

**Pat Riley (1993)**

Coaching a women's team to cohesion demands

- communicating frequently;
- the building of a social contract (core covenant);
- taking care when making changes;
- always explaining why actions are being taken;
- sharing ownership of as much planning as possible;
- keeping responsibilities as clear as possible;
- creating a psychologically stable environment;
- providing constant reassurance;
- celebrating all achievements, however small; and
- handling defeats and setbacks sensitively.

# The Four Steps to Team Building and Team Cohesion

Coaches need an appreciation of the process of building a team from birth to maturity and the relative roles of task and social cohesion at each stage of the journey. B.W. Tuckman (1965) developed the classic analysis of the four steps to building a team:

*1. Forming*   Individuals are gathered together and asked to commit to a common purpose.

*2. Storming* As the coach shapes the team, tension and conflict develop as players compete for selection, specific roles, and status.

*3. Norming* Conflicts begin to be resolved, and players accept their roles and commit to the team identity.

*4. Performing* The team is now achieving, highly unified in purpose and able to overcome problems and setbacks by working and staying together.

Each stage is a vital step toward the final, difficult stage of achieving effective performance while keeping a squad of players involved and committed. A final stage in the team's life cycle occurs when it ages and its performance diminishes. The coach will then have to re-form the team.

Coaches and players can check their responsibilities in contributing to the process of team cohesion by examining tables 11.4, 11.5, 11.6 (page 182), and 11.7 (page 183). In these tables, the team-building structure of forming, storming, norming, and performing is followed, identifying important aspects of both task and social cohesion. Many coaches inherit teams who may be in any of the stages described. The tables can be of great help in assessing a team's present level of cohesion and what steps they might take to improve it.

### TABLE 11.4—Forming the Team

**Stage 1 Forming: A settling-in period.**

| Task cohesion | Social cohesion |
| --- | --- |
| Good initial player recruitment will accelerate progress. | Recruit players who have the experience or potential to become involved in a demanding team venture. |
| Staff should be selected for core job skills, skill in individual and team interaction, and problem solving. | Communication, the major problem initially, moves from formal and coach-led to informal and player-led. |
| Planning is everything. | First meeting, first impressions, and the skills of the coach are important in selling the challenge. |
| It is important to define the vision and mission clearly:<br>• This is where we want to go.<br>• We want you to be a part of it.<br>• We can do this together.<br>• It should be both challenging and fun. | An atmosphere of competitive tension will exist at this stage as players informally rank their ability levels. |
| Begin the process of communication and getting players to buy into shared ownership of achieving the vision. | Players may buy in at this stage, but personal agendas ("What's in it for me?") will still dominate over any team agenda. |
| Coaches do not offer too much input at this stage; it's a time for building informal social relationships. | Establish house rules to mark boundaries for behavior. |

## TABLE 11.5—Players Bid for Places on the Team

**Stage 2 Storming: Players find their place, role, and status within the team.**

| Task cohesion | Social cohesion |
|---|---|
| The staff are role models, and they must stay strong in this difficult period. | This is an emotional time for players as they discover their allotted role and status within the team. |
| The team plan is now taking shape with specific objectives and identification of players for different roles and responsibilities. | With the internal competition for places comes the threat of<br>• power struggles in the leadership vacuum,<br>• formation of cliques and rivalries,<br>• anticoach attitudes, and<br>• noncommunication from the disaffected. |
| Coaches must ensure that everyone has a role and then persuade the player to buy into the plan. | A number of players will accept and identify with the roles allocated and will begin to move from a personal agenda to a team agenda, from "me" to "we." |
| Coaches must manage emotional reactions and tensions and must maintain a high level of communication through regular, relevant team meetings and one-on-one counseling. | Star players may seek special treatment. |
| Coaches must focus on the controllables and manage the team environment to minimize disturbance and distraction. | Players will establish informal networks of communication. |
| Coaches review and redefine each player's role as far as possible to create a working win-win situation. | Coaches should be careful with shared room allocations. |
| Coaches either manage or lose the rebels. | Players' individual personalities will emerge, and coaches will begin to see who will be high maintenance and who will be low maintenance. |
| The team begins to build its image—name, dress, and so forth. | At this stage players need help from coaches or counselors in order to become more self-aware and to understand others. |

## TABLE 11.6—The Team Norms and Sets Aside Differences

**Stage 3 Norming: Players start to take responsibility and perform their roles, and the team takes shape.**

| Task cohesion | Social cohesion |
|---|---|
| The mission statement or covenant—"the way we will do things as a team"—is agreed on. | Players have a good understanding of the coaches' philosophy and tactics and their specific roles. |
| Relevant, regular practice defines the way the team wants to play and begins to develop these elements:<br>• Clarity of tactics and roles<br>• Well-understood routines<br>• Specific job descriptions for individual players<br>• Heavy focus on common goals<br>• Strong team work ethic<br>• Agreed-on working procedures<br>• Improved team balance with better role integration | Through the physical proximity of practice, a social structure emerges:<br>• A captain is chosen.<br>• Team leaders develop.<br>• The pecking order of ability becomes clear.<br>• Friendship bonding occurs.<br>• Players now give and receive help. |
| Coaches must provide constant reinforcement and high levels of feedback. | The superordinate goal of beating the opposition creates unity behind a common purpose. |
| Coaches must logically match objectives to potential if there is a discrepancy; weaknesses must not be covered up. | Players are now willing to conform, balancing their individual needs with the needs of other team members. |
| Coaches must be proactive in dealing with the hot spots (team problems) and empower players in agreeing to the solution. | Players display greater appreciation and respect for the various roles on the team. |
| Coaches should sell, not yell, and maintain high levels of communication and sharing with the players. | Confidence improves, and the players learn to change negatives into positives. |
| Coaches must develop a professional environment with minimal distractions and disruptions. | Players accept greater accountability for their contribution to the team. |
| | Special care must be given to anyone still isolated at this stage. |
| | Family and friends are taken care of so they can fully support the player. |

## TABLE 11.7—The Team Performs With Cohesion

**Stage 4 Performing: The team cooperates to achieve competition goals.**

| Task cohesion | Social cohesion |
| --- | --- |
| The team is now tightly organized and structured. | The team is now beginning to feel distinctive, and players are committed to its development. |
| Coaches and players are fully committed. | Each player accepts his role and responsibility to<br>• put the team first,<br>• sacrifice when necessary,<br>• be prepared to help teammates,<br>• socialize with the team,<br>• conform to team rules, and<br>• accept valid criticism. |
| Coaches provide strong leadership. | Intrinsic motivation is high, and players are glad to be a part of this team. |
| Coaches keep the vision in front of the players. | Trust and honesty are high. |
| Coaches appreciate individual effort but reward the team for any success. | Players are coping better with emotional lows—nonselection, injury, and so forth. |
| Continuity of selection helps stability. | The development process has left players mentally tougher to deal with the unexpected dilemmas of the game. |
| A cooperative but competitive tension exists. | Victory or defeat will not disrupt cohesion. |
| Coaches now understand how to motivate each player. | Players are fully accountable for their actions, and the price of failure is high. |
| Coaches will keep listening to players, especially senior players, so they don't miss mood changes or other developments. | Some players may not have bonded—players from different cultures, new players, injured players. The team and coaches must cooperate to remedy this. |
| The team will now have a culture that will allow it to survive setbacks, learn from them, let go, and move on. | |
| Coaches must remain proactive and deal with problems early. | |
| Coaches will avoid overtraining and remember the value of fun as a way to influence mood. | |
| New recruits must be checked carefully to protect the team ethos. | |
| Everyone must keep learning. | |

# Summary

A group of players becomes an effective team when the coach creates a mission and environment that encourages the players to unite to achieve their goals by working together cohesively. This is a great coaching challenge, and success in building and maintaining team cohesion separates the great, the good, and the not-so-good coaches.

Cohesion begins with a vision that the whole team can believe in and a team image that is worth belonging to. The coach, then, must underpin these with the strong foundations of task cohesion and social cohesion. Soccer clubs at a recreational level might prioritize social cohesion, but clubs who intend to achieve at higher levels must drive task cohesion with social cohesion as a valuable by-product.

Players are challenged to be both part of task cohesion, knowing and doing their jobs well, and social cohesion, being able to integrate and contribute to team relationships. Coaches of women's teams are urged to understand the importance of social cohesion—described as a social contract of belonging and togetherness—that underpins all efforts to build task cohesion and then team cohesion. The importance of a coach's emotional intelligence is stressed as key to the maintenance of team cohesion over the season.

Finally, teambuilding, task cohesion, and social cohesion are combined in the four classic stages of forming, storming, norming, and performing.

A Japanese proverb can summarise this chapter: "None of us are as smart as all of us."

# CHAPTER 12

# Coaching: Creating the Future

Leadership is not really about leading;
It's about having guys follow you.
They make the choice.

**Steve Young, former quarterback, San Francisco 49ers**

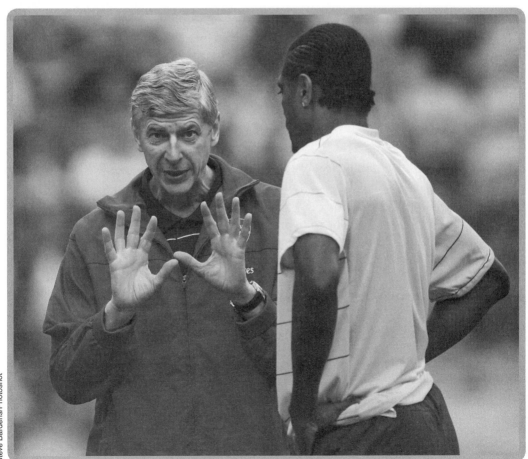

Steve Bardens/Photoshot

This book has consistently honored the tradition of coaching, the great coaches, and the importance of the coach–player relationship. This relationship is always based on the dynamic interchange of

- developments in the way the game is played,
- the motivation and personality of the player, and
- the personality and style of the coach.

The purpose of this book is to make coaches aware that the traditional coach–player relationship is changing and to offer them a range of new skills that allow them to get the best out of the modern player in the modern game. Sports always reflect the wider society, and now coaches are faced with players who present very different problems. Previously, coaches could assume motivation and attitude, and focus on developing their players' talent. With the modern player, the coaches must first of all win the battle of player attitude before they can begin to develop potential for the game.

Soccer is not the only ticket in town for this generation, and young players will reject soccer coaches and programs that do not meet their wider needs and life patterns. Many young people do not have a straight-forward passage through life, operate within a multi-agenda program, and are beset with a variety of influences. Their relationship to peers will be important, but they may not necessarily be team-oriented and could have difficulties with authority, discipline, and commitment. When retiring from college soccer, coach Rick Burns reflected on his coaching career, he spoke sincerely about his difficulties with the present generation of young players:

> Their neediness was energy sapping. Their fear of holding teammates accountable and their lack of courage to think and act independently were discouraging as well. Some of my players took the long route to adulthood. All of them are too young to know how little they know. (2008, 53)

As the evolution of the modern coach will always follow the evolution of the modern player, this book emphasizes that coaches must adapt to meet the new challenge. There is much that is good in present coaching styles and methods, but it is true that soccer tradition and culture, especially in Britain, have created a standard coaching philosophy based on domination, power, and authority. However, the circumstances that permitted autocratic leadership and a command–response culture have changed, and young players are more attuned to more democratic leadership and a consensus culture. Coaches must adapt. The key change that is stressed throughout this book is the need for coaches to sell their program—enthusing, involving, and engaging their players in the journey to soccer excellence—rather than yell and use their authority to impose their view of every situation. Table 12.1 offers coaches a chance to reflect on how they could adapt their style from traditional to modern.

| TABLE 12.1—The Move From Traditional to Modern Coaching | |
|---|---|
| **Traditional** | **Modern** |
| Focused on winning | Focused on winning (no change) |
| Task-centered | Player-centered |
| Results-dominated | Excellence-dominated |
| Instinctive | Careful planning |
| Player-dependent | Coach-influenced |
| Isolated | Mentored |
| "Me" | "We" |
| Authoritarian | Democratic |
| Yells | Sells |
| Speaks | Listens and then speaks |
| Trainer | Teacher |
| Ex-player | Qualified coach |
| Hard worker | Smart worker |

I once asked Bolo Zenden, a highly intelligent player who starred at Middlesbrough FC in the English Premier League, what he needed from his coach, and he gave this interesting response:

- Knowledge—an expert who understood his talent and could make him a better player
- Communication—someone who would share information freely and on his wavelength
- Belief—a coach who could convince him of the right way to play
- Openness—a willingness to listen, share views, and understand feelings
- Intelligence—to know when to drive hard and when to relax
- Trust—the strength to know when to stand back, let him play, and forgive his mistakes.

Table 12.2 (page 188) gives coaches a chance to assess themselves on their progress as modern coaches. Coaches must be brutally honest in their responses and be able to identify at least three pieces of supportive evidence. Any statement that cannot be answered "strongly agree" or "agree" must be cause for reflection, analysis, and discussion with fellow coaches or senior players.

## TABLE 12.2—Where Are You Now? A Coach's Self-Evaluation

| | Decide where you stand on the following questions and ✓ the box that best fits. | Strongly agree | Agree | Maybe | Disagree | Strongly disagree |
|---|---|---|---|---|---|---|
| 1. | Everyone knows how passionate and committed I am to coaching soccer. | | | | | |
| 2. | My personality and behavior always reflect a positive model to my players. | | | | | |
| 3. | I have clear goals and am tough enough to drive the program forward. | | | | | |
| 4. | I am a good communicator and always get my message across. | | | | | |
| 5. | Players enjoy playing for me. | | | | | |
| 6. | I have a clear understanding of how to develop players and teams. | | | | | |
| 7. | My strength is being able to plan, organize, and coach practice well. | | | | | |
| 8. | I have a good track record of identifying and recruiting talent. | | | | | |
| 9. | I am tactically sound and can teach a variety of formations. | | | | | |
| 10. | I coach game day well and always give my team the best chance to win. | | | | | |
| 11. | I pride myself on developing positive and productive relationships with players. | | | | | |
| 12. | Players who have played for me will say I got the best out of them. | | | | | |
| 13. | As far as possible I always try to share ownership with the players. | | | | | |
| 14. | I communicate constantly with the players, but especially I listen. | | | | | |
| 15. | The power of my player relationships is shown by their motivation to play. | | | | | |

From B. Beswick, 2010, *Focused for Soccer, Second Edition* (Champaign, IL: Human Kinetics).

# Coaching the Complete Player

The key lesson of this book is that performance follows attitude, and therefore, for coaches to develop complete players, they must coach attitude as well as talent. Not only does the coach still have to prepare a coaching program to meet the physical, technical, and tactical needs of a fast-changing, sophisticated game but they will have to increasingly act as psychologist in order to get engagement, commitment, and learning from their players. Players' attitudes, and whether they define any particular soccer situation they find themselves in positively or negatively, are derived from

- their own unique personalities;
- the influence of the significant people in their life, including the coach; and
- the impact of the coaching environment at their club.

This background defines the strategies open to the coach who wishes to develop complete players and shape attitudes in a positive way. Coaches can shape attitudes by incorporating 10 key strategies into their everyday coaching style:

1. Communicate more—this includes listening—with each player and not just the stars.
2. Build an ongoing relationship with each player; appreciate individual feelings and learn to assess mood.
3. Understand each player's personality and the best approaches for a positive response.
4. Be the model every day for the attitude and behavior you wish the players to follow.
5. Sell more and yell less; players need to be engaged and willing before they will commit.
6. Share ownership of the journey; it's about where the players want to go.
7. Make the player's significant family and friends part of the solution, not the problem.
8. Create a motivational coaching environment where players are challenged but always enjoy their soccer.
9. Develop a range of coaching strategies that can change a player's or team's attitude from negative to positive.
10. Create emotional stability—a defeat is only an opportunity lost! Learn but move on.

If performance follows attitude for the individual player, it also follows for the team; shaping team attitudes and managing team mood is a key element of successful coaching. The good coaches can prepare and manage a team for a game, but the great coaches prepare and manage teams successfully over a long and challenging season—and in the case of Sir Alex Ferguson, the manager of Manchester United, over 20 seasons!

In supporting the head coaches of Premier League soccer clubs, I saw my role including the following responsibilities:

■ Assessing the general mood or mind-set of the playing squad and coaching staff every day. A winning mind-set would reflect confidence, enthusiasm, work ethic, togetherness, willingness to learn, and so on. When these were missing, alarm bells rang.

■ Observing individual players for any recognizable changes in attitude or behavior. Attitude can change so quickly in young players faced with difficult challenges, in soccer and at home, and picking up early signs could help us be proactive in our response.

■ Reviewing the planning, preparation, and proposed program for the day and looking for potential negatives that could create anxiety, especially the key attitude killers of overtraining or overcoaching. While the coaches focused on the mechanics of the day, I would empathize with the players and try to judge their reaction. Coaches often changed direction after the potential player reaction to their plans was pointed out.

■ Checking all communication with the players to ensure positive messages and full understanding. Recently a Premier League manager was so disgusted at his team's first half performance, he conducted his half-time meeting on the field in front of the disgruntled fans. The team lost the game and then had a disastrous run of defeats. Coaches must be careful with what, when, where, and how they communicate with the team.

■ Advising the head coach when a strategy was needed to move the team or a player from a state of anxiety to a state of confidence. When our Brazilian midfielder, Juninho, was having a poor run of form, I suggested to Coach Steve Round that we cut a highlight film of Juninho's best moments playing for us and leave it in his locker. He was back to his best in the following game!

■ Dealing with any critical incident so that a positive mind-set was restored as quickly as possible. There will be thunderbolts in any challenging soccer season, and the key always is to avoid reacting emotionally but rather immediately begin dealing with the setback in a positive way that allows the team to move on quickly.

Of course, coaches without the help of sport psychologists must learn to be a little bit more of a psychologist and a little less of a trainer. It begins with learning to observe the players and team as people with feelings that can easily change. It goes on to becoming player-centered in planning, preparation, and organization, ensuring the players' needs are prioritized.

## Tosh Changes His Team From Anxious to Confident

Tosh Farrell, coach of Everton's under-9 team, knew his team would be anxious before playing at home against the Liverpool under-9 team. These boys lived near each other, went to the same schools, their parents knew each other, and so on. Tosh knew the importance of the game would be blown out of all proportion, and anxiety could defeat his team—the better team in terms of soccer—and so he created a pregame strategy to relax the players and restore confidence.

When the players arrived in the dressing room pregame, Tosh sat down with them and asked who had watched the X-Factor (a TV talent show) the night before. Most had, so then Tosh checked who their parents had voted for. Tosh made fun of some of the decisions, and his warm personality and great sense of humor relaxed the players and took their focus and anxiety away from the game. Three minutes from kick-off, Tosh jumped up and led a good humored and confident team on the field and on to a 7-1 victory!

Then it is building positive and strong player relationships. Finally it means developing a range of strategies that can respond to negative situations and maintain player and team confidence and self-belief.

## The Coach as a Model

It has been said that coaches get the players they deserve, and it is true that the presence and personality of the leader has a very great influence on the followers. So, to some extent, coaches dictate the team attitudes by their appearance, personality, and behavior. I do like to ask coaches the question:

Would you like to play for you?

Successful coaches have

- presence and impact—they must appear and act like a leader at all times;
- expertise that players respect because they know it can improve their game;
- vision and purpose, a clear plan for success that they sell to their players;
- courage, the determination to stick to the plan when setbacks occur;
- optimism, a constant belief that good preparation will lead to eventual success;

- communication skills that every day gets the right message across;
- relationship skills that make players feel special, cared for, and inspired;
- emotional intelligence that deals with negatives and allows the team to stay in the positive;
- calmness: regardless of the circumstances, the coach stays a panic-free zone; and
- composure—always bigger than any one game, the coach does not let any one result affect overall progress.

One of the ways in which players' behavior is shaped is by imitation of those they admire. It is clear that if a coach can integrate these very positive characteristics into her everyday coaching style, then the rewards will be players who reflect those strengths.

# The Coach as a Teacher

To build a successful team the coach must teach and develop at every opportunity

1. the physical, technical, and tactical capacity to deliver the performance required; and
2. the attitude in practice and games that underpins the emergence of mentally tough performance.

Lee Carsley, whose story is told in chapters 1 and 2, had talent but not attitude. Once he developed a winning attitude, his talent flourished, and

## THE SEVEN HABITS OF "LUCKY" COACHES

1. They have a **positive** outlook on life.
2. They **position** themselves to be lucky; they stay in the game.
3. They have a sound coaching **philosophy** but are flexible.
4. They are **proactive;** they make things happen.
5. They stay in **control;** they lead from the front.
6. They focus on **relationships;** they know their players well.
7. They work **hard and smart.**

*It's funny; the harder I practice, the luckier I get.*

**Gary Player, golf champion**

he performed excellently for 15 years in the English Premier League. Good coaches teach their players to do simple things well, by habit, and in the critical moments of the game. They create a learning environment that is focused, purposeful, and varied but also challenging:

- The coaches challenge the players constantly.
- The players are encouraged to challenge each other.
- Most importantly, the players must challenge themselves.

Good coaches do not necessarily need to teach competitive and winning attitudes separately but rather as an integral part of their soccer club's daily existence and work. Players carry their off-the-field attitude on to the field, so coaches need to instill firm guidelines that help players acquire the necessary self-discipline of a winning attitude. So for Lee Carsley, building a winning attitude meant

- being on time,
- not forgetting anything,
- being fully prepared for practice or game,
- looking smart,
- being enthusiastic,
- being a good team member,
- being first on the field,
- being last off the field,
- trying hard at all practices,
- listening to and learning from the coach,
- helping set things up and put things away,
- being competitive at all times,
- always trying to be the best,
- being a positive substitute,
- congratulating other players,
- being able to deal with mistakes and recover,
- being first at practice after a defeat,
- being loyal to the team, and
- challenging teammates to be better.

Teaching these elements requires coaches who are willing to set guidelines, observe player responses, and correct as appropriate. When coaches insist on the above from an early age, they are actually beginning the process of self-discipline that is crucial to the players who will finish as top performers and professionals. Equally important, coaches are helping this challenged generation emerge as better adults and citizens.

Good coaches reinforce their messages on winning attitudes and behavior by using a variety of audio visual aids. Personal reminder cards (see the Sunderland example on page 195), photographs, wall posters, visiting speakers, and film clips are some of the methods available. Characteristics of the learning environment that I have helped encourage at top soccer clubs include the following:

- A clear sense of purpose: everything is designed to help achieve the vision.
- The engagement of the players: they are always given a reason why we are practicing or playing in a particular way.
- Clear instruction: players need to know clearly what the coach requires of them.
- The importance of hard work: repetition, but with variety, thus avoiding boredom.
- Best practice images: the players constantly see film clips that emphasize the excellence being sought.
- Attitude-shaping: every practice situation is coached as a mental and emotional challenge as well as a physical, technical, and tactical challenge.
- Reinforcement: good attitudes and behavior are noted and rewarded.
- Feedback: the coach's job is to constantly show players how they can improve.
- Expertise: when players need extra help or a specialist's help, it is provided whenever possible.

## The Coach and Relationships

The coach has to lead and manage by building relationships that motivate and drive their staff and players to be the best they can be. Such relationships are now built on selling rather than yelling and are much more likely to involve the players in the ownership of the process. Dr. Martyn Newman describes three conditions for establishing social relationships:

**1.** Relationships work best when people are recognized and treated as equals.

**2.** People willingly collaborate when they see benefits for themselves.

**3.** People work best when they own the relationships by having the freedom to contribute to it.

Newman goes on to sum up: "Engaging with people as partners enables you to adopt an approach that rewards wins, positive interactions, and sustainable relationships" (2007, 134).

## SHAPING GAME CONFIDENCE

Below is a reprint of the card that every young player at Sunderland Football Club's academy must carry with him and read before games. This trigger card is the coaches' way of programming their players' minds to be positive, at the time when they are most vulnerable to the negative.

### Game Confidence and Self-Talk: Read Before Every Game

- I am still willing to work hard.
- I trust the coaches because they trust me.
- I am as ready as I'll ever be for this game.
- I will take responsibility for my game and my decisions, good or bad.
- I always play hard and accept knocks as part of the game.
- I may make mistakes, but I know how to recover.
- If I miss a shot, I will get the next one.
- If we are losing, I will work even harder.
- I love the club and feel proud to wear the shirt.
- We are tough and hard to beat as a team.

*We are a team!*

Such relationships will not be successful unless the coach has built a high level of trust with the players, often called social capital. Social capital is built or destroyed everyday by the quality and sincerity of the coach's interactions with the players. Coaches build social capital by

- winning respect for their expertise—the players know the coach can take them where they want to go;
- clarity of direction—the players are never confused as to what is required of them;
- communication, inspiration, and persuasion—the players believe the message;
- shared values—the coach operates under a value system the players will buy into;
- emotional stability—the players respect the way the coach handles the bad times;
- warmth of personality, humor—the players enjoy the presence of the coach;
- caring for the players as people—the players know they will always receive help with personal problems;

- trust—players know that what the coach says will happen, does happen!
- honesty—players know that the coach will be honest with them, even when giving the bad news; and
- fairness—the coach might not treat all players the same (in our professional world, we prioritize players according to their contribution to our success), but there will be an essential fairness of approach.

If a coach builds a reserve of social capital with a squad, there is a greater likelihood of being forgiven for a mistake and also of being given a greater extent of goodwill in times of adversity.

## New Leaders in Soccer

The modern coach this book describes is an expert at both production—organizing, teaching, and driving the physical, technical, and tactical elements of the game—and relationships—getting the best out of players and teams. The challenge and fun of coaching is that it demands the rational analysis and logic of the scientist but also the empathy and instinct of an artist. While all coaches start their career fully focused on production, it is true that most coaches end their careers absorbed in the power of relationships and attitude. Both are essential to peak performance:

Good production + good relationships = peak performance

Good production + poor relationships = potential to win but little commitment

Poor production + good relationships = commitment to win but little ability

This chapter has focused on the importance to the coach of building positive relationships that can act as the glue that cements their players to the cause and binds them together as a team. Such positive relationships create resonance—an environment where players feel their feelings are being taken care of—as distinct from dissonance—a feeling of not being cared for.

Players would describe a coach capable of creating resonance as upbeat, warm, caring, approachable, a good listener, tuned in to emotions, genuinely interested in the players, optimistic, humorous, and secure in themselves. On the other hand, players would describe a dissonant leader as irritable, touchy, domineering, cold, pessimistic, governed by fear or ego, short-sighted, and captive to their own emotions. As the mind-set of the players is largely determined by the personalities and actions of the coaches

## THE FOUR GREAT DEMANDS OF MODERN COACHING

**1.** A sophisticated understanding of the game and a willingness to stay a student of the game

**2.** The presence, personality, and communication skills to sell players the dream of winning

**3.** The intellectual ability to cope with ever-increasing performance analysis—sport science, psychology, and match analysis—and to use it to make better decisions

**4.** The emotional intelligence to stay stable and balanced and maintain healthy relationships with players, manage their feelings, and release their emotional power.

and the coaching environment, it is clear that coaches must develop a new range of relationship skills:

- Being emotionally intelligent, learning to be in tune with both themselves and their players
- Creating resonance, a positive emotional climate that frees the best in players
- Preventing dissonance by planning, organizing, and behaving in a way that minimizes negatives
- Communicating sensitively, knowing that when leaders speak, their words and actions have a strong emotional impact on the team
- Engaging players by creating a motivational coaching environment that recruits players to the cause
- Providing emotional leadership by guiding the players feelings through the emotional roller-coaster of the season

Figure 12.1 (page 198) guides coaches through the process they must manage to develop emotional leadership skills.

Paul Barron, goalkeeping coach at Newcastle United, is an advocate of relationship coaching and once described his philosophy as

They forget what you say to them.
They forget what you do with them.
But they never forget how you made them feel!

Relationship coaching is about coaches connecting with their players, getting to the real pulse of the team, and releasing a powerful collective emotional energy. This very often is the edge that allows teams to survive the bad times and go on to remarkable achievements.

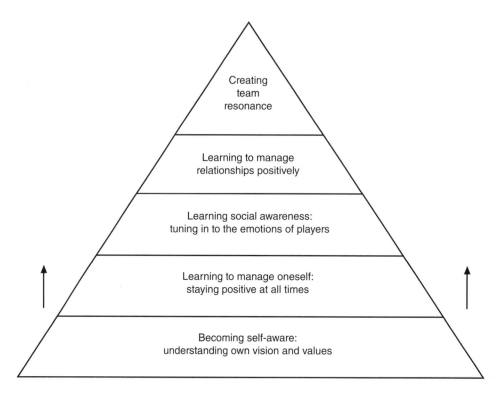

FIGURE 12.1   The route to resonant and emotionally intelligent leadership.

# Summary

This chapter ends the book by emphasizing the crucial importance to the player and the team of experienced, intelligent, and thoughtful coaching. Coaching is always a challenge but never more so than now when young players can be much more difficult to engage and teach. To overcome this, coaching has to become more an exercise in shared ownership, player-centered, and with coaching styles directed more to selling than yelling.

Earlier in the book the concept of the complete player is explained, and coaches are urged to understand their crucial role in shaping the attitudes of their players and teams. Creating a confident and competitive mind-set in very challenging game situations is a key coaching skill, and coaches must develop a number of strategies for moving negative attitudes back into the positive.

The coach is reminded that younger players especially learn attitude and behavior by imitating role models, and the coach is a very important model in the life of a young player. Part of the responsibility of coaching and leadership is setting the example every day in all aspects of high performance for players to follow. This is why it is said that coaches eventually finish with the players they deserve.

Coaches are also reminded of the importance of their role as teachers, not only of soccer techniques and systems, but also of player attitudes. Good coaches establish a learning environment where clear guidelines are set, standards imposed and monitored, feedback given, and players learn to accept responsibility.

The modern coach understands the power of relationships and works every day to build up social capital to strengthen the bonds between coach and player, coach and coach, and player and player. These strong relationships, based on a sense of working and caring for each other, are the glue that holds the team together when in a slump and drives them forward toward achievement.

The new leaders in soccer will be influenced and shaped more and more by their emotional intelligence and their understanding of the psychology of players and performance. They will go beyond coaching the physical, technical, and tactical elements of the game to get the best out of the players and team both mentally and emotionally. Such new leaders will demonstrate mature emotional intelligence and the ability to create a resonant coaching environment.

Many teams are now prepared well physically, technically, and tactically, so the coach who can shape attitudes positively and release the power of positive emotions is the coach who will find the winning edge.

# References

Balague, G. 2007. Three perspectives on female motivation. *Championship Performance* 11, (128):2.

Barrell, J., and D. Ryback. 2008. *Psychology of champions.* Westport, CT: Praeger.

Bradley, B. 1998. *Values of the game.* New York: Artisan.

Bull S., and C. Shambrook. 2004. *Soccer: The mind game.* Ramsbury: The Crowood Press.

Burns, R. 2008. No job for old men: A mini memoir. *Coach and Athletic Director* 78 (December):52-57.

Carragher, J. 2008. *Carra: My autobiography.* London: Bantam Press.

Courtenay, B. 1989. *The power of one.* London: Heineman-Mandarin.

Covey, S.R. 1989. *The 7 habits of highly effective people.* New York: Simon and Schuster.

Dale, G., and S. Conant. 2004. *101 teambuilding activities: Ideas every coach can use to enhance teamwork, communication and trust.* Distributed by Excellence In Performance.

DeBoer, K. 2004. *Gender and competition: How men and women approach work and play differently.* Monterey: Coaches Choice.

DiCicco, T., C. Hacker, and C. Salzberg. 2002. *Catch them being good: Everything you need to know to successfully coach girls.* New York: Viking.

Gilbert, R. 2006. *Read this book tonight to help you win tomorrow.* Charlotte, NC: Championship Performance.

Gilbourne, D. 1999. *Insight: The Football Association Coaches Journal* 2:37.

Goldberg, A.S. 1997. *Playing out of your mind.* Spring City, PA: Reedswain.

———. 1998. *Sports slump busting.* Champaign, IL: Human Kinetics.

Goleman, D. 1995. *Emotional intelligence.* London: Bloomsbury.

———. 1998. *Working with emotional intelligence.* London: Bloomsbury.

———. 2002. *The new leaders.* London: Little, Brown.

Green, E., and A. Green. 1977. *Beyond biofeedback.* New York: Dial Press.

Gucciardi, D.F., S. Gordon, and J. Dimmock. 2008. Towards an understanding of mental toughness in Australian football. *Journal of Applied Sport Psychology* 20 (3):261-81.

Gyp, P. 1998. Getting players to take psychological responsibility. *FIFA.com. [online].* 15 paragraphs. Available: www.fifa.com/newscentre/news/newsid = 71559.html [December 21, 2009].

Halberstam, D. 1999. *Playing for keeps: Michael Jordan and the world he made.* New York: Random House.

Holtz, L., and J. Heisler. 1989. *The fighting spirit: A championship season at Notre Dame.* New York: Pocket Books.

Isberg, L. 1997. *Insight: The Football Association Coaches Journal* 1:16.

Jackson, P., and H. Delehanty. 1995. *Sacred hoops: Spiritual lessons of a hardwood warrior.* New York: Hyperion.

Jenner, B. and M. Seal. 1996. *Finding the champion within: A step-by-step plan for reaching your full potential.* New York: Simon and Schuster.

Johnson, M.D. 1996. *Slaying the dragon: How to turn your small steps to great feats.* New York: ReganBooks.

Johnson, M.E. 2007. Coaches corner. *Championship Performance* 11 (128): 1.

Jordan, M. and M. Vancil. 1994. *I can't accept not trying: Michael Jordan on the pursuit of excellence.* New York: Harper Collins.

Kanter, R.M. 2004. *Confidence: How winning streaks and losing streaks begin and end.* New York: Crown Business.

Kipling, R. 1895. *The Second Jungle Book.* London: Macmillan and Co.

Kramer, J. 1970. *Lombardi: winning is the only thing.* New York: World.

Lavin, J. 2005. *Management secrets of the New England Patriots.* 2 vols. Stamford, CT: Pointer Press.

Loehr, J.E. 1994. *The new toughness training for sports.* New York: Plume.

Loehr, J.E., and P.J. McLaughlin. 1990. *Mental toughness training.* Chicago: Nightingale Conant (audio cassette).

Lombardi, V. 1996. *Coaching for teamwork: Winning concepts for business in the twenty-first century.* Bellevue, WA: Reinforcement.

Marano, H. E. 2008. *A nation of wimps: The high cost of invasive parenting.* New York: Broadway.

Michels, R. 1996. Team-Building. Presented at the 2nd European Coaches Convention. U.E.F.A. Lecture Series No. 2.

Miller, B. 1997. *Gold minds.* Ramsbury: The Crowood Press.

Morris, T., and J. Summers. 1995. *Sports psychology: Theory, applications, and issues.* Queensland: John Wiley.

Nelson, M.B. 1998. *Embracing victory: Life lessons in competition and compassion.* New York: Morrow.

Newman, M. 2007. *Emotional capitalists: The new leaders.* Monterey: Coaches Choice.

Parcells, B. 1995. *Finding a way to win: The principles of leadership, teamwork, and motivation.* New York: Doubleday.

Pitino, R., and P. Forde. 2008. *Rebound rules: The art of success 2.0.* New York: Harper Collins.

Pitino, R. and B. Reynolds. 1997. *Success Is a choice: Ten steps to overachieving in business and life.* New York: Broadway.

Ravizza, K., and T. Hanson. 1995. *Heads up baseball: Playing the game one pitch at a time.* Indianapolis: Masters Press.

Reardon, J. 1998. Sports psychology and soccer. Presentation given at the Sportsmind Conference, Warrington, England.

Riley, P. 1993. *The winner within: A life plan for team players.* New York: Putnam's Sons.

Shula, D., and K. Blanchard. 1995. *Everyone's a coach: You can inspire anyone to be a winner.* Grand Rapids, MI: Zondervan.

Smith, E. 2008. *What sport tells us about life: Bradman's average, Zidane's kiss and other sporting lessons.* London: Viking.

Taylor, J. 1998. Focus and Intensity for Training and Competition. Presentation at 1998 conference of the Association for the Advancement of Applied Sports Psychology, Vancouver, BC.

Taylor, J., and D. Wilson, eds. 2005. *Applying sports psychology: Four perspectives.* Champaign, IL: Human Kinetics.

Thompson, J. 1995. *Positive coaching: Building character and self-esteem through sports.* Portola Valley, CA: Warde.

Tuckman, B.W. 1965. Development Sequence in Small Groups. *Psychological Bulletin* 63: 384-399.

*USA Today.* 2004. 10 Toughest Athletes Case Study. February.

Voight, M. 2008. *Mental toughness training for soccer: Maximizing technical and mental mechanics.* Monterey: Coaches Choice.

Walsh, B. 2009. *The score takes care of itself: My philosophy of leadership.* New York: Penguin.

Walsh, B., B. Billick, J. Peterson, and NetLibrary, Inc. 1998. *Finding the winning edge.* Champaign, IL: Sports Publishing (electronic book).

Whitaker, D. 1999. *The spirit of teams.* Ramsbury: The Crowood Press.

Wise, M. 2008. *Championship Performance.*

Wooden, J. 1972. *They call me coach: As told to Jack Tobin.* Waco, TX: Word Books.

# Index

*Note:* The italicized *f* and *t* following page numbers refer to figures and tables, respectively.

# About the Author

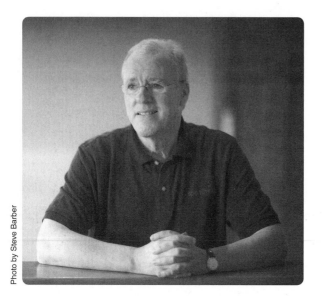

Photo by Steve Barber

**Bill Beswick** is a leader in the field of sport psychology and is especially known for his work with professional soccer teams. He has a master's degree, five years of experience as head coach of England's men's basketball team, and substantial experience in teaching, lecturing, and coaching, all of which make him ideally suited as the first full-time sport psychologist in English professional soccer. From 1996 to 1999 Beswick helped Derby County Football Club compete in the world's toughest league, the English Premier League. He then took a job with Manchester United, perhaps the world's best-known soccer club. There he worked with players and coaches to build mental toughness and competitiveness in an environment where the team is expected to win every time it takes the field.

When Manchester United and England assistant coach Steve McClaren was appointed manager of Middlesbrough Football Club in 2001, he surprised the soccer world by appointing Beswick as his assistant manager, the most senior role for a sport psychologist in the history of British soccer. For five seasons Beswick supported McClaren during Middlesbrough's most successful period in history. From 2006 to 2007 Beswick was psychologist with England's national men's team. Following a spell at Sunderland FC, Bill at present provides specialist advice to clubs in England, Holland, and the United States. While continuing to develop Sportsmind Ltd., a company that has provided sport psychology services and resource materials to coaches and athletes for more than 20 years.